STRATEGIES and INTERVENTIONS to REDUCE SUICIDE

PROCEEDINGS OF A WORKSHOP

Alexandra Andrada, Sharyl J. Nass, and Joe Alper, *Rapporteurs*

Forum on Mental Health and Substance Use Disorders

Board on Health Care Services

Board on Health Sciences Policy

Health and Medicine Division

The National Academies of
SCIENCES · ENGINEERING · MEDICINE

THE NATIONAL ACADEMIES PRESS
Washington, DC
www.nap.edu

THE NATIONAL ACADEMIES PRESS   500 Fifth Street, NW   Washington, DC 20001

This activity was supported by Purchase Order No. 75FCMC19P0036 with the Centers for Medicare & Medicaid Services and Contract No. HHSN263201800029I, Order No. HHSN26300025 with the National Institutes of Health and by the American College of Clinical Pharmacy, American Psychiatric Nurses Association, American Psychological Association, Association for Behavioral Health and Wellness, Council on Social Work Education, Janssen Research & Development, LLC, National Academy of Medicine, National Institute on Alcohol Abuse and Alcoholism, National Institute on Drug Abuse, Office of the Assistant Secretary for Planning and Evaluation, Optum Behavioral Health, Think Bigger Do Good Policy Series (a partnership of the Scattergood Foundation, Peg's Foundation, Patrick P. Lee Foundation, and Peter & Elizabeth Tower Foundation), U.S. Department of Veterans Affairs, and Well Being Trust. Any opinions, findings, conclusions, or recommendations expressed in this publication do not necessarily reflect the views of any organization or agency that provided support for the project.

International Standard Book Number-13: 978-0-309-27773-0
International Standard Book Number-10: 0-309-27773-6
Digital Object Identifier: https://doi.org/10.17226/26471

Additional copies of this publication are available from the National Academies Press, 500 Fifth Street, NW, Keck 360, Washington, DC 20001; (800) 624-6242 or (202) 334-3313; http://www.nap.edu.

Copyright 2022 by the National Academy of Sciences. All rights reserved.

Printed in the United States of America

Suggested citation: National Academies of Sciences, Engineering, and Medicine. 2022. *Strategies and interventions to reduce suicide: Proceedings of a workshop*. Washington, DC: The National Academies Press. https://doi.org/10.17226/26471.

The National Academies of
SCIENCES • ENGINEERING • MEDICINE

The **National Academy of Sciences** was established in 1863 by an Act of Congress, signed by President Lincoln, as a private, nongovernmental institution to advise the nation on issues related to science and technology. Members are elected by their peers for outstanding contributions to research. Dr. Marcia McNutt is president.

The **National Academy of Engineering** was established in 1964 under the charter of the National Academy of Sciences to bring the practices of engineering to advising the nation. Members are elected by their peers for extraordinary contributions to engineering. Dr. John L. Anderson is president.

The **National Academy of Medicine** (formerly the Institute of Medicine) was established in 1970 under the charter of the National Academy of Sciences to advise the nation on medical and health issues. Members are elected by their peers for distinguished contributions to medicine and health. Dr. Victor J. Dzau is president.

The three Academies work together as the **National Academies of Sciences, Engineering, and Medicine** to provide independent, objective analysis and advice to the nation and conduct other activities to solve complex problems and inform public policy decisions. The National Academies also encourage education and research, recognize outstanding contributions to knowledge, and increase public understanding in matters of science, engineering, and medicine.

Learn more about the National Academies of Sciences, Engineering, and Medicine at **www.nationalacademies.org**.

The National Academies of
SCIENCES • ENGINEERING • MEDICINE

Consensus Study Reports published by the National Academies of Sciences, Engineering, and Medicine document the evidence-based consensus on the study's statement of task by an authoring committee of experts. Reports typically include findings, conclusions, and recommendations based on information gathered by the committee and the committee's deliberations. Each report has been subjected to a rigorous and independent peer-review process and it represents the position of the National Academies on the statement of task.

Proceedings published by the National Academies of Sciences, Engineering, and Medicine chronicle the presentations and discussions at a workshop, symposium, or other event convened by the National Academies. The statements and opinions contained in proceedings are those of the participants and are not endorsed by other participants, the planning committee, or the National Academies.

For information about other products and activities of the National Academies, please visit www.nationalacademies.org/about/whatwedo.

PLANNING COMMITTEE FOR A WORKSHOP ON STRATEGIES AND INTERVENTIONS TO REDUCE SUICIDE[1]

MARY ROARY (*Co-Chair*), Director, Office of Behavioral Health Equity, Office of the Intergovernmental and External Affairs, Substance Abuse and Mental Health Services Administration
MATTHEW TIERNEY (*Co-Chair*), President, American Psychiatric Nurses Association; Clinical Professor, University of California, San Francisco, School of Nursing; Clinical Director of Substance Use Treatment and Education, University of California, San Francisco, Office of Population Health
ERIN BAGALMAN, Director, Division of Behavioral Health Policy, Office of the Assistant Secretary for Planning and Evaluation, U.S. Department of Health and Human Services
MICHAEL F. HOGAN, Principal, Hogan Health Solutions LLC
ANDREW MOON, Associate Director, Education and Training, Suicide Prevention Program, Office of Mental Health and Suicide Prevention, U.S. Department of Veterans Affairs
JANE PEARSON, Special Advisor to the Director on Suicide Research, National Institute of Mental Health

Project Staff

ALEXANDRA ANDRADA, Director, Forum on Mental Health and Substance Use Disorders, and Program Officer
ADRIENNE FORMENTOS, Research Associate (*from July 2021*)
ANESIA WILKS, Senior Program Assistant
SHARYL NASS, Senior Director, Board on Health Care Services
ANDREW M. POPE, Senior Director, Board on Health Sciences Policy

Consultant

JOE ALPER, Consulting Writer

---

[1] The National Academies of Sciences, Engineering, and Medicine's planning committees are solely responsible for organizing the workshop, identifying topics, and choosing speakers. The responsibility for the published Proceedings of a Workshop rests with the workshop rapporteurs and the institution.

FORUM ON MENTAL HEALTH AND SUBSTANCE USE DISORDERS[1]

COLLEEN L. BARRY (*Co-Chair*), Johns Hopkins Bloomberg School of Public Health
HOWARD H. GOLDMAN (*Co-Chair*), University of Maryland School of Medicine
MARGARITA ALEGRÍA, Harvard Medical School
ERIN BAGALMAN, Office of the Assistant Secretary for Planning and Evaluation, U.S. Department of Health and Human Services
CARLOS BLANCO, National Institute on Drug Abuse, National Institutes of Health
DARLA SPENCE COFFEY, Council on Social Work Education
CHRIS M. CROWE, U.S. Department of Veterans Affairs
W. PERRY DICKINSON, University of Colorado
SYLVIA K. FISHER, Health Resources and Services Administration
RICHARD G. FRANK, Harvard Medical School
PAMELA GREENBERG, Association for Behavioral Health and Wellness
KRISTIN KROEGER, American Psychiatric Association
HUSSEINI K. MANJI, Janssen Research and Development, LLC
R. KATHRYN McHUGH, Harvard Medical School and Mclean Hospital
BEN MILLER, Well Being Trust
ANNIE PETERS, National Association of Addiction Treatment Providers
KATHY PHAM, American College of Clinical Pharmacy
JOE PYLE, Scattergood Foundation
DEIDRA ROACH, National Institute on Alcohol Abuse and Alcoholism, National Institutes of Health
MARY ROARY, Substance Abuse and Mental Health Services Administration
MARTIN ROSENZWEIG, Optum Behavioral Health
GLORINDA SEGAY, Indian Health Service
RUTH SHIM, University of California, Davis
MATTHEW TIERNEY, University of California, San Francisco, School of Nursing and Office of Population Health *(representing the American Psychiatric Nurses Association)*

---

[1] The National Academies of Sciences, Engineering, and Medicine's forums and roundtables do not issue, review, or approve individual documents. The responsibility for the published Proceedings of a Workshop rests with the workshop rapporteurs and the institution.

Reviewers[1]

This Proceedings of a Workshop was reviewed in draft form by individuals chosen for their diverse perspectives and technical expertise. The purpose of this independent review is to provide candid and critical comments that will assist the National Academies of Sciences, Engineering, and Medicine in making each published proceedings as sound as possible and to ensure that it meets the institutional standards for quality, objectivity, evidence, and responsiveness to the charge. The review comments and draft manuscript remain confidential to protect the integrity of the process.

We thank the following individuals for their review of this proceedings:

CRYSTAL L. BARKSDALE, National Institute of Mental Health
ANNA FERRERAS, National Academies of Sciences, Engineering, and Medicine
JANE PEARSON, National Institute of Mental Health

Although the reviewers listed provided many constructive comments and suggestions, they were not asked to endorse the content of the proceedings nor did they see the final draft before its release. The review of this proceedings was overseen by **HUGH TILSON,** University of North Carolina. He was responsible for making certain that an independent examination of this proceedings was carried out in accordance with the standards of the National Academies and that all review comments were carefully considered. Responsibility for the final content rests entirely with the rapporteurs and the National Academies.

---

[1] This text was changed after prepublication release.

Acknowledgments

The National Academies of Sciences, Engineering, and Medicine's Forum on Mental Health and Substance Use Disorders wishes to express its sincere gratitude to the planning committee co-chairs Mary Roary and Matt Tierney for their valuable contributions to the development and organization of this workshop. The forum wishes to thank all of the members of the planning committee, who collaborated to ensure a workshop complete with informative presentations and rich discussions. Finally, the forum wants to thank the speakers and moderators, who generously shared their expertise and their time with workshop participants.

Support from the many sponsors of the Forum on Mental Health and Substance Use Disorders is critical to the forum's work. The sponsors include the American College of Clinical Pharmacy, American Psychiatric Nurses Association, American Psychological Association, Association for Behavioral Health and Wellness, Council on Social Work Education, Janssen Research & Development, National Academy of Medicine, National Institute on Alcohol Abuse and Alcoholism, National Institute on Drug Abuse, Office of the Assistant Secretary for Planning and Evaluation, Optum Behavioral Health, Think Bigger Do Good Policy Series (a partnership of the Scattergood Foundation, Peg's Foundation, Patrick P. Lee Foundation, and Peter and Elizabeth Tower Foundation), U.S. Department of Veterans Affairs, and Well Being Trust. We also thank staff member Ana Ferreras for reading and providing helpful comments on this manuscript.

Contents

ACRONYMS AND ABBREVIATIONS	xvii
PROCEEDINGS OF A WORKSHOP	1
OVERVIEW OF THE WORKSHOP	1
SUICIDE TRENDS IN U.S. SUBGROUPS	2
OPPORTUNITIES IN HEALTH CARE TO REDUCE SUICIDE RISK	19
EXPERIENCES IN IMPLEMENTING SUICIDE PREVENTION CARE IN FEDERAL HEALTH CARE SETTINGS	21
Assessment and Management of Those at Risk for Suicide, 21	
PROMOTING LETHAL MEANS SAFETY AMONG VETERANS: OPPORTUNITIES AND CHALLENGES	23
SUICIDE PREVENTION AND CARE PROGRAM	26
IMPROVING SUICIDE PREVENTION: ADDRESSING KNOWN BARRIERS TO HEALTH CARE ACCESS	28
IMPROVING SUICIDE PREVENTION: ADDRESSING KNOWN BARRIERS TO HEALTH CARE ACCESS FOR LGBTQIA+ PEOPLE IN INSTITUTIONAL SETTINGS	29
RISK ID: THE VA SUICIDE RISK IDENTIFICATION STRATEGY	35
SUICIDE PREVENTION: BARRIERS TO CARE AMONG BLACK YOUTH AND FAMILIES	37
SUICIDE PREVENTION: STIGMA AND THE COVID-19 PANDEMIC	39

LEVELS OF PROGRESS TOWARD PREVENTION	41
BUILDING 9-8-8: AN OPPORTUNITY TO BUILD INCLUSIVE CARE STRUCTURES	42
IMPROVING CARE COORDINATION WITHIN CRISIS SERVICES	42
THE 9-8-8 LIFELINE: POTENTIAL AND IMPLICATIONS FOR CRISIS RESPONSE	43
The Community Mental Health Services Framework, 43	
Effectiveness of National Crisis Lines, 45	
Veterans Crisis Line 9-8-8 Expansion Initiative and Implications, 47	
9-8-8 ROLLOUT: PRIVACY, CONFIDENTIALITY, AND EQUITY CONSIDERATIONS	48
The 9-8-8 Workforce and Culturally and Linguistically Appropriate Services, 48	
PATIENT-CENTERED CARE CONSIDERATIONS IN CRISIS SERVICES FOR AMERICAN INDIAN/ALASKA NATIVE PEOPLE	50
BUILDING EQUITY INTO THE FRONT END OF 9-8-8	51
BUILDING CULTURAL COMPETENCE WITHIN CRISIS SERVICES	54
A Potential Framework for Developing Culturally Responsive and Personalized Evidence-Based Mental Health Interventions for Culturally Diverse Populations, 54	
BEYOND CULTURAL COMPETENCY	55
WORKING IN DIVERSE COMMUNITIES	56
LATINX YOUTH AND THE UNDOCUMENTED	57
BUILDING CULTURAL COMPETENCE WITHIN CRISIS SERVICES	59
9-8-8, HEALTH EQUITY, AND FAITH WITHIN THE BLACK COMMUNITY	59
A HISTORIC FIRST: SPECIALIZED SERVICES IN 9-8-8 FOR LGBTQIA+ YOUTH	61
ENSURING 9-8-8 SERVES ALL	61
INCLUDING SCHOOLS IN THE CRISIS RESPONSE SYSTEM	62
DISCUSSION: HEALTH EQUITY AND 9-8-8	63
REFLECTIONS: OPPORTUNITIES TO BUILD INCLUSIVE CARE STRUCTURES	64
REFERENCES	66
APPENDIX A STATEMENT OF TASK	75
APPENDIX B WORKSHOP AGENDA	77
APPENDIX C SPEAKER AND MODERATOR BIOGRAPHIES	87

Boxes, Figures, and Table

BOXES

1 Observations and Suggestions Made by Individual Workshop Participants, 3
2 Research Opportunities Available at NIMH, 19
3 Key Features of the Zero Suicide Initiative, 27

FIGURES

1 Age-adjusted suicide mortality in the United States, 1999–2019, 10
2 Suicide rates in U.S. youth ages 10 to 19 years old, 1999–2018, 11
3 U.S. youth suicide rate by gender, 1999–2018, 11
4 Age-adjusted suicide rates by race, 1999–2019, 12
5 Suicide rates in U.S. youth ages 10 to 19 years old by ethnicity, 2010–2019, 12
6 Age-adjusted suicide rates in the United States by state, per 100,000 individuals, 2019, 13
7 Comparison of suicide incidence rates between Black and White youth from 2001 to 2015, 14
8 Suicide rates by age and sex for U.S. children and adolescents, 2015–2019, 15
9 Percentage of U.S. high school students reporting suicidal thoughts and behavior in the past 12 months by sexual identity, 2019, 15

10 The role of firearms and other lethal means in suicides for veterans and nonveterans, 23
11 Emotional dysregulation can affect some people more than others when they respond to a stressful event, 29

TABLE

1 Minimum Screening Requirements by Setting for Risk ID, 36

Acronyms and Abbreviations

ASL	American Sign Language
ASQ	Ask Suicide-Screening Questions
C-SSRS	Columbia-Suicide Severity Rating Scale
CDC	Centers for Disease Control and Prevention
CLAS	Culturally and Linguistically Appropriate Services
CPR	cardiopulmonary resuscitation
CSRE	VA Comprehensive Suicide Risk Evaluation
EHR	electronic health record
FCC	Federal Communications Commission
HHS	U.S. Department of Health and Human Services
IHS	Indian Health Service
IRR	incidence rate ratio
LGBTQIA+	lesbian, gay, bisexual, transgender, queer and/or questioning, intersex, and asexual and/or ally
LOG	natural logarithm
MIRECC	Mental Illness Research, Education, and Clinical Center

NIMH	National Institute of Mental Health
NOSI	Notice of Special Interest
PICOT	Population, Intervention, Comparison or Control, Outcome, and Time Period
QPR	question, persuade, and refer
Risk ID	VA Suicide Risk Identification Strategy
SA/SI	suicide attempt/suicide ideation
SAMHSA	Substance Abuse and Mental Health Services Administration
SWAT	Special Weapons and Tactics
TTY	teletypewriter
VA	U.S. Department of Veterans Affairs

Proceedings of a Workshop

OVERVIEW OF THE WORKSHOP[1]

Reducing suicide-related mortality is a global imperative declared by the World Health Organization (WHO, 2014). The persistent trends in suicide necessitate action among mental health care providers and payers, researchers, and community leaders. The suicide prevention movement has been gaining momentum as organizations, advocates, and others have increasingly collaborated on effective strategies. Health care settings provide an important opportunity for suicide intervention and prevention, but they cannot yet fully manage suicide risk because of a lack of training, knowledge gaps, and reimbursement challenges. School, workplace, and community-based interventions can help reduce the incidence of suicidal behavior, as can better access to care and reduced access to lethal means of suicide (Hogg et al., 2021; National Action Alliance for Suicide Prevention, 2017; Pistone et al., 2019).

To better understand the strategies to improve access to effective interventions to prevent suicide, the Forum on Mental Health and Substance Use Disorders at the National Academies of Sciences, Engineering, and Medicine hosted a two-part virtual public workshop, Strategies and Interventions to

---

[1] The planning committee's role was limited to planning the workshop, and the Proceedings of a Workshop was prepared by the workshop rapporteurs as a factual summary of what occurred at the workshop. Statements, recommendations, and opinions expressed are those of individual presenters and participants, and are not necessarily endorsed or verified by the National Academies of Sciences, Engineering, and Medicine, and they should not be construed as reflecting any group consensus.

Reduce Suicide, on June 22, 2021, and July 28, 2021. The presentations and discussions during the first webinar on June 22 examined the scope of the public health problem, discussed the implementation of effective approaches for suicide prevention care, and addressed the known barriers to health care access. The second webinar on July 28 focused on building 9-8-8, the new nationwide emergency number designated to the National Suicide Prevention Lifeline, and participants discussed current crisis systems, gaps, challenges, and needs for marginalized populations. Appendix A contains the workshop Statement of Task, and Appendix B contains the workshop agendas, respectively.[2] Appendix C contains biographical sketches of the speakers and the moderators of the workshop. The objectives of the workshop were to discuss:

- The scope of the public health problem, with a focus on data regarding suicidal ideation, suicide attempts, and death by suicide;
- What is known about the effectiveness of approaches and interventions to reduce harm and prevent risk of suicide;
- Policy opportunities to support, improve, and implement early interventions to increase access and quality of care for individuals at risk of suicide; and
- Areas where further evidence or attention is needed to improve the quality of care available across the continuum for suicide prevention.

This Proceedings of a Workshop summarizes the presentations and discussions. The speakers, panelists, and workshop participants presented a broad range of views and ideas. Box 1 presents an overview of observations and suggestions from individual presentations and discussions and are discussed throughout the proceedings.

SUICIDE TRENDS IN U.S. SUBGROUPS

To provide context for the workshop, Jeffrey A. Bridge,[3] director of the Center for Suicide Prevention and Research at Nationwide Children's Hospital, and Crystal L. Barksdale, acting deputy director and chief of Minority Mental Health Research for the Office for Disparities Research and Workforce

---

[2] For additional information, see https://www.nationalacademies.org/event/06-10-2021/integrating-serious-illness-care-into-primary-care-delivery-a-workshop-first-webinar (accessed October 25, 2021) and https://www.nationalacademies.org/event/10-26-2020/integrating-serious-illness-care-into-primary-care-delivery-a-workshop#sectionEventMaterials (accessed October 25, 2021).

[3] Complete titles and affiliations for all speakers are available in Appendix C.

BOX 1
Observations and Suggestions Made by Individual Workshop Participants

Suicide Trends in U.S. Subgroups
- Overall, suicide was the 10th leading cause of death in the United States in 2019, accounting for 47,500 deaths. (Bridge)
- From 1999 to 2019, suicide rates among American Indian and Alaska Natives children and adolescents were significantly higher than among any other racial subgroup in the United States. (Bridge)
- Colorado Children's Hospital has declared a state of emergency because of the rising number of young people presenting to the emergency department with suicidal thoughts or behaviors. (Bridge)
- The National Violent Death Reporting System has begun capturing information about sexual identity and sexual orientation, which will make it possible going forward to understand at a regional or national level some of the factors associated with suicide by sexual orientation or sexual identity status. (Bridge)
- At the same time the COVID-19 pandemic was raging, the United States was experiencing other upheavals, particularly the racial awakening typified by the Black Lives Matter movement. This confluence of events has likely had an outsized effect on Black children and adolescents and highlights the need for culturally sensitive adaptations of effective interventions to address the problem of suicide among Black youth. (Bridge)
- Mental health care services are a critical component of suicide prevention efforts, and those services addressing suicide prevention can occur in a variety of settings, including crisis centers, health centers, clinics, in the home, and other locations specific to the population. (Barksdale)
- Reasons for underuse of mental health services vary among racially and ethnically diverse groups and individuals in the LGBTQIA+ community, but some of the most cited reasons include stigma surrounding seeking help, structural inequalities in the mental health care service system, and limited knowledge of and access to resources. Other reasons include the limited availability of culturally and linguistically competent or culturally appropriate services and limited mental health literacy. (Barksdale)

continued

BOX 1 Continued

- There is a pressing need to have layered suicide prevention approaches that include policies and protocols for workflow; training; developmentally timed, layered, evidence-based practices; coordination across systems of care; and better use of data for action. (Wilcox)
- The Garrett Lee Smith Campus Suicide Prevention Grant Program should become an ongoing program and not merely discretionary with regard to federal budgeting. (Hogan, McKeon)
- Schools can be an important component of upstream interventions. Having a defined pathway for referrals into treatment would make it easier for schools and other screening settings to be part of an integrated system of care. (Wilcox)

Experiences in Implementing Suicide Prevention Care in Federal Health Care Settings
- VA developed the 2019 clinical practice guidelines through a process of assembling multidisciplinary experts using the Population, Intervention, Comparison or Control, Outcome, and Time Period (PICOTS) framework. This created 22 recommendations to put the best clinical evidence into clinical practice. (Brenner)
- Lethal means safety is an intentional, voluntary practice to reduce access to lethal methods of suicide in order to reduce suicide risk. This can be accomplished using a cable lock to secure a firearm, storing a firearm or ammunition outside of the home, or keeping medications in a secure lockbox stored away from those in a household who are at risk of suicide. (Simonetti)
- Lethal means safety counseling is not a single intervention, but rather needs to be provided across many different settings and through different messengers delivering different messages to a heterogeneous mix of at-risk populations. (Simonetti)
- Research is needed to understand the perspectives of people who own firearms based on other characteristics such as gender and experiences with racial discrimination or trauma. (Simonetti)
- Within the Indian Health Service (IHS), the Suicide Prevention and Care program operates in conjunction with programs in mental health and substance use disorders and with the IHS Telebehavioral Health Center of Excellence to provide programs to tribal communities and tribal nations that focus on behavioral health care and suicide prevention. (End of Horn)
- The Zero Suicide model is a comprehensive approach to care that aims to reduce the risk of suicide for all individuals seen in health

care systems through the use of seven essential elements for patient safety—lead, train, identify, engage, treat, transition, and improve. The Zero Suicide pilot model is set to end in 2021. (End of Horn)
- Future plans within IHS include using crisis lines to assist with follow-up contacts, using case managers to conduct continual tracking of patients in care pathways, and to enhance the functionality of electronic health records by adding alerts and establishing data-sharing agreements. (End of Horn)

Improving Suicide Prevention: Addressing Known Barriers to Health Care Access
- Based on feedback from those who have had a personal experience related to suicide, language should shift from using the term *committed suicide* to *died by suicide* or *died of suicide*, and from *dealing with* suicidal patients to *working with* them. (Whiteside)
- Schools can establish safe spaces and social groups on campus that promote school connectedness among LGBTQIA+ students, a major protective factor against suicidal behaviors. Schools can also adopt inclusive curricula that do not neglect LGBTQIA+ health concerns and that foster mental health literacy. They can also vet community care providers and confirm they are knowledgeable about and provide supportive care to LGBTQIA+ people. (Willging)
- Primary care clinics should increase outreach efforts in the communities they serve, transitioning to gender-neutral restrooms, and displaying artwork and educational materials that signify a welcoming environment. Clinics can also start collecting and using data on gender identity and sexual orientation as part of routine clinical care and make it possible for staff to understand and address disparities affecting LGBTQIA+ patients. (Willging)
- The U.S. Department of Veterans Affairs' (VA's) Suicide Risk Identification Strategy Program (Risk ID) is a national standardized process for suicide risk screening using high-quality, evidenced-based tools and practices to facilitate and encourage fidelity to best screening and evaluation practices. (Brenner)
- Two broad factors contribute to barriers to care among Black youth. One relates to stigma associated with mental illness and service use, and the primacy of family support; the other is the frequent misinterpretation of presenting symptoms in schools. (Lindsey)

continued

BOX 1 Continued

The 9-8-8 Lifeline: Potential and Implications for Crisis Response
- Congress passed the National Suicide Hotline Designation Act of 2020, known colloquially as the 9-8-8 Act. As a result, in 2022, dialing 9-8-8 from any phone line, (mobile phone, landline, or Voice over Internet Protocol line) will connect the caller with the National Suicide Prevention Lifeline. (Everett)
- The 9-8-8 system will build on the structure of the National Suicide Prevention Lifeline, which since 2005 has used the number 1-800-273-TALK (1-800-273-8255). Unlike 9-1-1 calls, 9-8-8 calls will all be directed to this national structure instead of being dispatched locally. (McKeon)
- Upon reaching 9-8-8, callers will hear a recorded message telling them to "press 1" if they are calling about a veteran or service member, which will then connect them to the veterans crisis line, or "press 2" if they need to be connected to a crisis counselor who is fluent in Spanish. Otherwise, the call will be distributed to one of the 184 local crisis centers located in every one of the 50 states as well as the territory of Guam. If the call is not answered within the first couple of minutes, it will go to a backup center—this is a feature that is not part of that 9-1-1 system. In addition, it will feature a text chat service. (McKeon)
- A study showed that crisis line callers who spoke with a trained counselor, had a significant reduction in risk from the beginning to the end of the call. (Gould)
- Lifeline services now have evolved to include a crisis chat and intervention feature. Two-thirds of individuals who use the chat function reported that the chat was helpful and were significantly and substantially less distressed at the end of the chat intervention than they were in the beginning. (Gould)
- Ongoing evaluation has shown that callers were over five times more likely to have less distress at the end of the call than at the beginning and were almost five times more likely to have less suicidal ideation at the end of the call than the beginning. Callers were 91 percent less likely to have suicidal urgency at the end of the call than at the beginning, and 83 percent of callers reported feeling better following their call. (Kearney)

9-8-8 Rollout: Privacy, Confidentiality, and Equity Considerations
- There is concern regarding the implementation of 9-8-8. Call volume could drastically increase with the ease of the three-digit number, which is good in terms of accessibility, and possibly

- decreased stigma, but more services will need to be in place. When the full range of options is not available, the result is overreliance on 9-1-1, often with individuals ending up in jail, the emergency department, or the morgue. (O'Brien)
- The key to success with the 9-8-8 rollout will be providing callers with access to the full continuum of care so they receive the right type and amount of care. (O'Brien)
- To improve equity, it is imperative to leverage a well-trained, diverse, and even nonclinical workforce, including peer-support specialists. (O'Brien)
- The IHS emphasizes humanization in health care through a person-centered approach that asserts the intrinsic dignity of all human beings and by adopting the core values of honesty and integrity, caring compassion, altruism, empathy, and respect for others. (End of Horn)
- Implementing the 9-8-8 system creates an opportunity to build a more equitable and responsive system that is not only evidence based and evidence informed but informed by the community and individuals' lived experience. (Armstrong, Johnson)
- The challenge is to seize the opportunity afforded by the 9-8-8 rollout to work with community partners and community media to create grassroots messaging that can educate communities, combat stigma, and address concerns about receiving mental health treatment; to use expertise and care providers of color who have traditionally served historically marginalized communities, often without access to government grants and contracts, and engaging them in the planning; and to give voice to those with lived experience. (Armstrong)

Building Cultural Competence Within Crisis Services
- The PersIn Approach to developing personalized, evidence-based interventions for culturally diverse populations entails three steps: identifying factors and understanding potential dimensions upon which personalization for culturally diverse populations may need to occur. When assessing risk and protective factors for suicidal behavior, it is important to account for cultural factors such as family conflict, social discord, acculturative stress, minority stress, cultural sanctions related to suicide, and idioms of distress. (Yeh)
- Results of the PersIn Approach gives service providers a sense of the factors that may be especially important to address with a particular individual before they begin the intervention. The goal is to provide a culturally responsive intervention that accounts for impor-

continued

BOX 1 Continued

tant cultural dimensions while making it possible to standardize the delivery of tools and personalize the intervention to an individual when implemented. (Yeh)
- Cultural competency is not a clinical skill. Rather, it is an opportunity for individuals to learn about local customs and local perspectives, to build networks, and to incorporate those elements and aspects into the care that is provided and allow the care to be responsive to the community needs. (End of Horn)
- A significant part of planning for the 9-8-8 rollout includes having conversations about equity, such as how to handle calls from a non-native English speaker and where the responsibility of the 9-8-8 system morphs into the community's responsibility to provide language assistance. (Battle)
- Critical race theory, a methodology for helping investigators maintain consciousness of racialized constructs and historical sociopolitical mechanisms, can help investigators and practitioners understand the unique experiences of individuals. (Chávez)
- Latino Critical Theory allows investigators to examine how multiple forms of oppression can intersect with the lives of people of color and how interactions manifest in day-to-day experiences unique to the Latinx community, such as immigration status, language, ethnicity, and culture. (Chávez)
- Undocumented critical (UndocuCrit) theory offers a critical approach for analyzing how racist immigration practices, policies, and rhetoric function to spread fear among undocumented populations. (Chávez)
- In terms of suicide prevention efforts the focus should be on expanding social media campaigns to reduce the stigma of mental health and substance use and promote safety, as well as enforcing nondiscrimination laws, guaranteeing universal coverage for all youth, implementing trauma-informed policies, keeping families together, and promoting community resiliency. Promoting mental health from a young age should be emphasized and include anti-bullying training, and there should be an effort to highlight evidence-based practices for Latinx behavioral health and to create partnerships between family, community, and schools to promote resilience and heal trauma. (Chávez)
- SAMHSA, the National Institute on Minority Health and Health Disparities, and the Asian American Health Initiative in Montgomery County, Maryland, started a Healthy Mind Initiative that is reaching out to Asian communities to increase awareness and promote

suicide prevention among Asian adolescents. This initiative relies on individuals from the various communities who speak the language and understand the specific culture. This is the type of involvement that will be critical for implementing 9-8-8 initiatives. (Zhang)
- The rollout of the 9-8-8 system could address health equity issues by increasing access to mobile crisis teams for Black families, which in turn could save lives by avoiding engagement with law enforcement. (Johnson)
- Involving faith communities in suicide prevention efforts can help people get connected to services and coordinate their care, as well as help educate individuals about mental health and how it can affect them. (Johnson)
- 9-8-8 is a significant advance for high-risk populations because the legislation requires an implementation plan for "specialized services" for a variety of high-risk populations, including LGBTQIA+ youth, as well as minority and rural populations. This is the first and only time an LGBTQ-inclusive bill passed unanimously. (Brinton)
- The 9-8-8 initiative will neither be truly inclusive nor fully accessible unless text message and direct video call acceptance capabilities are integrated into the rollout. People with disabilities have to deal with multiple phone numbers. One important goal of the 9-8-8 rollout should ensure that everyone has only one number to remember and that it responds to text or video calls without any extra steps. (Schneider)
- It is imperative for the nation to build a universal behavioral health system for prevention, early identification, and intervention to minimize crises while also addressing the failings of the current crisis response system for children. (Hoover)
- The new National Center for Safe Supportive Schools, funded by SAMHSA, focuses on three areas: developing comprehensive school mental health systems, implementing culturally responsive and equitable policies, and supporting trauma-informed, healing-centered, practices. (Hoover)
- There are three levels of intervention strategies: those that can help prevent people from becoming suicidal in the first place, those that can prevent individuals who are having suicidal thoughts from progressing to an acute suicidal crisis, and those such as 9-8-8 that can help someone at imminent risk. (McKeon)
- Research on suicide gatekeeper skills include teaching diverse groups (e.g., school staff, co-workers) how to "question, persuade, and refer (QPR)" a person at risk. (Limandri)
- Family, friends, and neighbors are the most essential first responders in a suicide crisis. (Limandri)

Diversity at the National Institute of Mental Health (NIMH), presented some of the data on suicide rates for various populations in the United States.

Overall, suicide was the 10th leading cause of death in the United States in 2019, accounting for 47,500 deaths, said Bridge. Death by suicide spans all age groups, he explained, and it is the second leading cause of death among individuals ages 10 through 34. Data from the National Vital Statistics System show that age-adjusted suicide rates in the United States increased for both males and females from 1999 through 2019 (see Figure 1), with an overall increase of 35.2 percent (Hedegaard et al., 2021). There is a gender paradox regarding suicide and suicidal behavior in that suicide rates for males have remained four times higher than for women over that time span, while the rate of suicide attempts by young females is three to four times higher than by young males.

Suicide rates have shown to be persistent. Between 1999 and 2007, there was a decline among U.S. youth ages 10 to 19 years old, but since then, suicide rates increased by 88 percent between 2007 and 2018 (see Figure 2). Even accounting for a drop in suicides in 2019, the increase from 2007 would be approximately 80 percent. Broken down by gender, suicide rates for both females and males fell between 1999 and 2007, by 16 percent and 20 percent respectively, while from 2007 to 2018 the suicide rate among females in the 10- to 19-year-old population increased by 147 percent, compared to 75 percent in males in the same age group (see Figure 3). The larger increase among females contributed to a narrowing of the gender gap in this age range (Ruch et al., 2019), said Bridge.

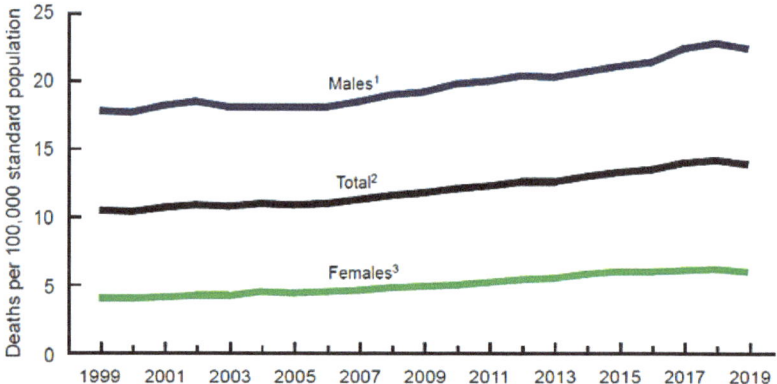

FIGURE 1 Age-adjusted suicide mortality in the United States, 1999–2019.
SOURCES: Presented by Jeffrey A. Bridge on June 22, 2021, at the workshop on Strategies and Interventions to Reduce Suicide; Hedegaard et al., 2021.

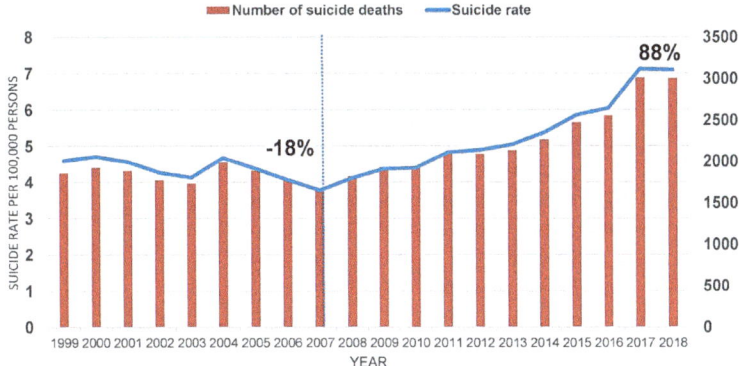

FIGURE 2 Suicide rates in U.S. youth ages 10 to 19 years old, 1999–2018.
SOURCES: Presented by Jeffrey A. Bridge on June 22, 2021, at the workshop on Strategies and Interventions to Reduce Suicide. Data from CDC, 2021a.

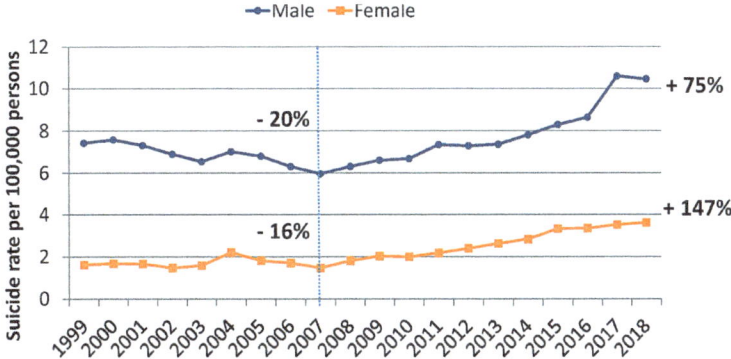

FIGURE 3 U.S. youth suicide rate by gender, 1999–2018.
SOURCES: Presented by Jeffrey A. Bridge on June 22, 2021, at the workshop on Strategies and Interventions to Reduce Suicide. Data from CDC, 2021a.

There are racial differences in U.S. suicide rates, Bridge continued, with suicide rates among White individuals across the life span being higher than among every other racial subgroup (see Figure 4). However, from 1999 to 2019, suicide rates among American Indian and Alaska Natives children and adolescents were significantly higher than among any other racial subgroup in the United States (see Figure 4). Moreover, suicide rates among children and adolescents ages 10–19 years were approximately 35 percent higher among American Indian and Alaska Native females compared to both Black and Asian and Pacific Islander males in the same age group, said Bridge. Parsing the data by ethnicity shows that suicide rates across all ages, including among

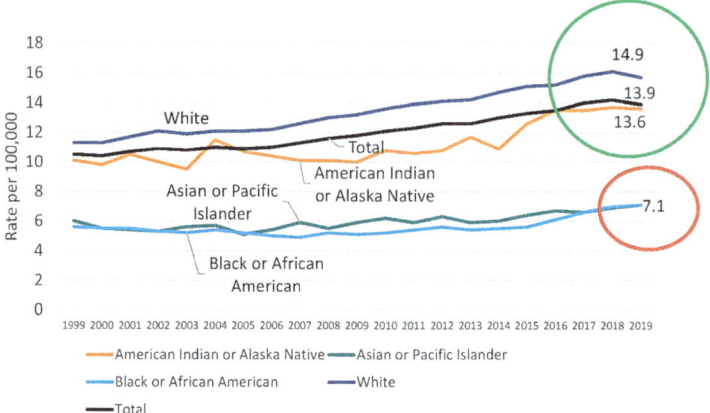

FIGURE 4 Age-adjusted suicide rates by race, 1999–2019.
SOURCES: Presented by Jeffrey A. Bridge on June 22, 2021, at the workshop on Strategies and Interventions to Reduce Suicide; Ramchand et al., 2021.

individuals ages 10 to 19 years old, are higher among non-Hispanic individuals, though the gap between non-Hispanic and Hispanic females ages 10 to 19 years old is small (see Figure 5).

Bridge described the geographic urban versus rural differences in suicide rates in the United States, as seen in Figure 6. He noted that while there would be some variation in the data over the past 20 years, the states with the highest suicide rates have remained unchanged. While there has been no published

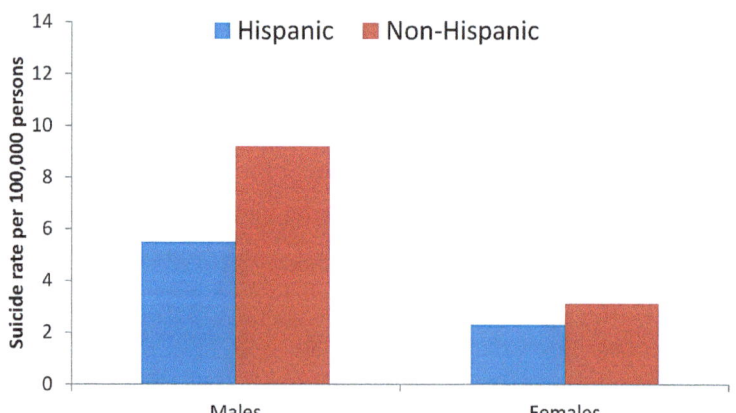

FIGURE 5 Suicide rates in U.S. youth ages 10 to 19 years old by ethnicity, 2010–2019.
SOURCES: Presented by Jeffrey A. Bridge on June 22, 2021, at the workshop on Strategies and Interventions to Reduce Suicide; CDC, 2021a.

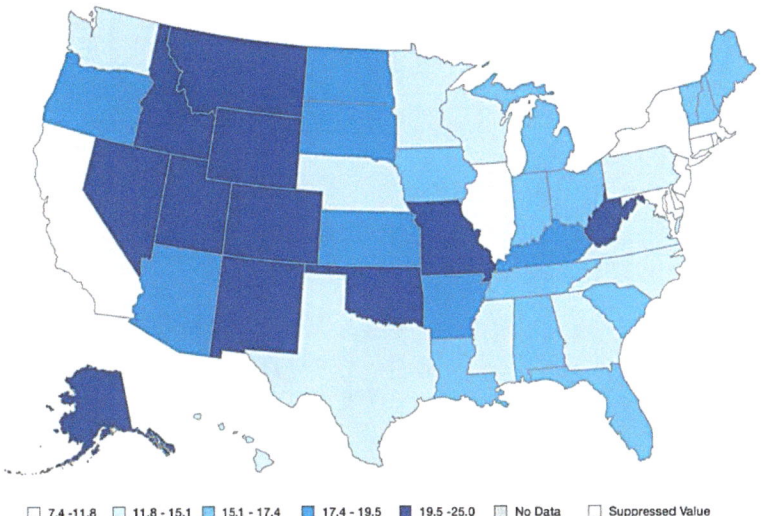

FIGURE 6 Age-adjusted suicide rates in the United States by state, per 100,000 individuals, 2019.
SOURCES: Presented by Jeffrey A. Bridge on June 22, 2021, at the workshop on Strategies and Interventions to Reduce Suicide; CDC, 2021a.

research examining the causes for these differences, people have proposed several explanations. One might be that higher suicide rates in the western United States are tied to a higher density of firearms among the population. Another explanation could be disparities in access to health care. "In my mind, it would be a good study to do to begin to understand the contributors to this geographic variation in suicide in the United States," said Bridge.

In 2015, Bridge and his team began looking at trends in suicide among children 5 to 11 years old in the United States and found that there was no trend overall. However, when his team stratified the data by race, they saw two divergent patterns. Among White children, and particularly 5- to 11-year-old boys, there was a significant decrease in the suicide rate from 2001 to 2015, while among Black children the opposite was true (Bridge et al., 2015, 2018). Extending the age range, Bridge and his team found that around age 13, the suicide rate among Black youth began to decrease relative to the rates among White youth, a decline that continued throughout adolescence (Bridge et al., 2015) (see Figure 7). He noted that suicide was the 16th leading cause of death among Black youth and the 12th leading cause of death among White youth in 1999, and by 2018 it had become the 7th leading cause of death for both Black and White youth.

Regarding nonfatal suicidal behavior, researchers have found that there was a decline in suicidal thoughts and behaviors across racial and ethnic groups

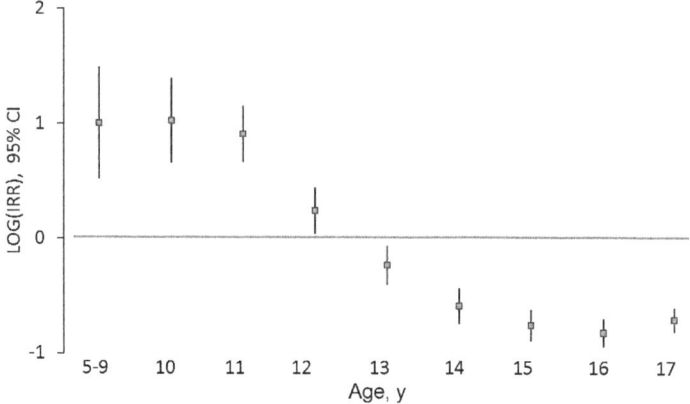

FIGURE 7 Comparison of suicide incidence rates between Black and White youth from 2001 to 2015.
NOTES: Blue squares indicate the estimated LOG of the age-specific IRR, vertical lines indicate 95% CI, and reference group is White youth. CIs of 95% that do not include zero are considered statistically significant. CI = confidence interval; IRR = incidence rate ratio; LOG = natural logarithm; y = years.
SOURCES: Presented by Jeffrey A. Bridge on June 22, 2021, at the workshop on Strategies and Interventions to Reduce Suicide; Bridge et al., 2018.

between 1991 and 2017 (Lindsey et al., 2019). However, when the researchers looked specifically at Black adolescents, there was a significant linear trend increase in the suicide attempt rate for both Black boys and Black girls. In particular, said Bridge, there was an increase for Black males in suicide attempts requiring medical treatment (CDC, 2019; Lindsey et al., 2019).

In preteens, suicide rates for both males and females are well under 1 per 100,000 persons through age 9 but begin to accelerate through adolescence (see Figure 8). For children ages 5 through 12, suicide deaths have increased by 280 percent since their low in 2008 (CDC, 2021a). One study found that 43.1 percent of suicide attempt and suicide ideation (SA/SI) visits were among children 5 to 11 years old (Burstein et al., 2019; Mishara and Stijelja, 2020). "This is a trajectory we do not want to see," said Bridge. Rates of youth ages 5 to 12 presenting to emergency care settings for self-harm have increased about 5-fold between 2001 and 2019 (CDC, 2021a). Bridge noted that the COVID-19 pandemic has exacerbated this situation to such a degree that Colorado Children's Hospital has declared a state of emergency because of the rising number of young people presenting to the emergency department with suicidal thoughts or behaviors (Children's Hospital Colorado, 2021).

In recent years, the National Violent Death Reporting System has begun capturing information about gender identity and sexual orientation, which will make it possible going forward to understand at a regional or national level some

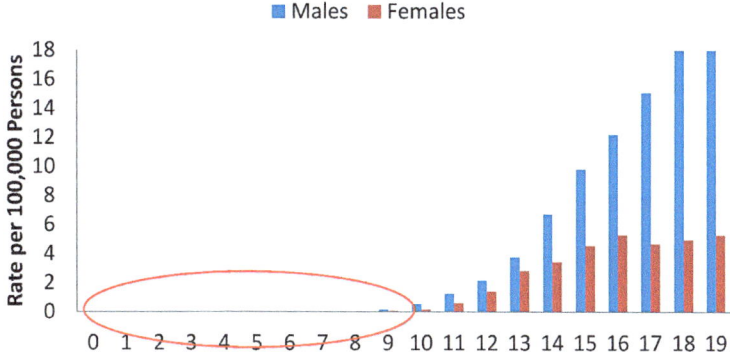

FIGURE 8 Suicide rates by age and sex for U.S. children and adolescents, 2015–2019.
SOURCES: Presented by Jeffrey A. Bridge on June 22, 2021, at the workshop on Strategies and Interventions to Reduce Suicide; CDC, 2021a.

of the factors associated with suicide by sexual orientation, or gender identity status (CDC, 2021b; Ream, 2020), which Bridge called a positive step forward. Data from the Centers for Disease Control and Prevention (CDC) Youth Risk Behavior Survey show that students identifying as lesbian, gay, or bisexual have the highest rates of thinking about, planning, and attempting suicide (CDC, 2019). The rates for those who identify as "not sure" and who may be questioning their sexual identity are also higher than for heterosexual students (see Figure 9). The same pattern exists for students who identify as having a same sex partner compared to those with an opposite sex partner only, added Bridge.

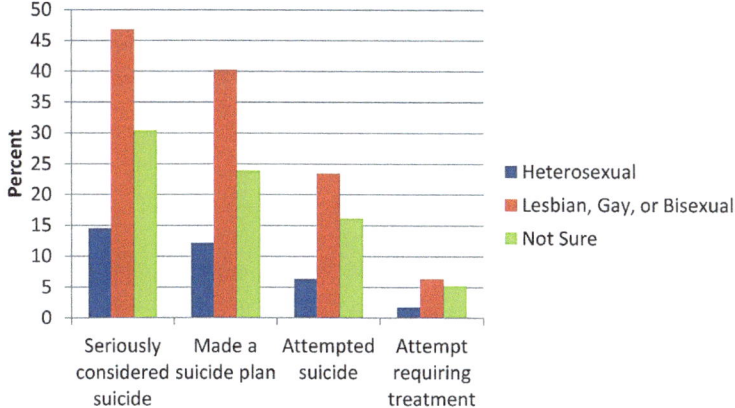

FIGURE 9 Percentage of U.S. high school students reporting suicidal thoughts and behavior in the past 12 months by sexual identity, 2019.
SOURCES: Presented by Jeffrey A. Bridge on June 22, 2021, at the workshop on Strategies and Interventions to Reduce Suicide. Data from CDC, 2019.

A divergent pattern was found between Black and White individuals between 2017 and 2020. When comparing the rates of death by suicide during two periods—March through May 2017 and March through May 2020—the rates for Blacks increased by 94.1 percent but decreased for Whites by 45.1 percent (Bray et al., 2021), though Bridge cautioned that the absolute numbers of deaths by suicide were small. In 2020, another study that examined suicidal ideation, anxiety symptoms, substance use, trauma, and stress-related symptoms found that there were disproportionate adverse mental health outcomes for younger adults, racial and ethnic minorities, essential workers, and unpaid adult caregivers (Czeisler et al., 2020).

At the same time of the COVID-19 pandemic, the United States was experiencing large public protests, particularly the racial awakening typified by the Black Lives Matter movement.[4] Bridge mentions these events due to the outsized effect on Black children and adolescents and highlights the need for culturally sensitive adaptations of effective interventions to address the problem of suicide among Black youth. As an example, Bridge described a promising intervention developed by researchers at DePaul University who adapted an existing cognitive-behavioral, group-based preventive intervention that aims to enhance adaptive coping skills and reduce suicidal ideation (Robinson et al., 2021). The adapted 15-session intervention incorporates strategies that counter stressors associated with systemic racism that burdens Black adolescents. The results look promising, Bridge noted, with the adolescents being favorable and receptive to this intervention, thus showing that it is feasible to implement.

Barksdale then discussed the current status of suicide prevention and use of mental health services among U.S. subpopulations. She began by explaining that NIMH is the lead federal agency for research on mental health disorders, supporting more than 3,000 research grants and contracts at universities and other institutions across the United States and abroad. In addition, NIMH's intramural program supports approximately 600 scientists.

Mental health care services, said Barksdale, are a critical component of suicide prevention efforts, and those services addressing suicide prevention can occur in a variety of settings, including crisis centers, health centers, clinics, in the home, and other locations specific to the population. For example older adults may use services at rehabilitation centers or nursing homes, and children and adolescents may be primarily served in schools. In fact, she added, suicide prevention requires the active engagement of multiple systems working in coordination across multiple settings, she said. Integrating suicide prevention into the delivery of mental health care services has been found to help prevent suicides (While et al., 2012), and this fosters a comprehensive

---

[4] See https://blacklivesmatter.com (accessed October 25, 2021).

approach to care by encouraging increased collaboration between and coordination of services among care providers.

However, individuals at risk for suicide—and particularly youth and historically minoritized populations—often do not seek mental health services (Hom and Stanley, 2021). This reality affects suicide prevention outcomes and exacerbates disparities in suicidal behavior and suicide prevention. For this reason, Barksdale noted, it is important to understand help-seeking behaviors in order to promote effective suicide prevention efforts and answer questions such as whether a person has or has not considered mental health care, whether they have sought advice from family and friends about getting care, and what their experience with the care they have received has been and if it helped them get better. "Overall, we want to provide and make available culturally and linguistically appropriate mental health care services that meet the needs of individuals at risk, and then encourage individuals to see these services as an option to address their needs," said Barksdale.

Turning to the subject of mental health services used by specific subpopulations, she said research suggests that across racial and ethnic groups, service use among youth at elevated risk for suicide is consistently below 50 percent (Michelmore and Hindley, 2012) and that only half of the youth (56.1 percent) discharged from inpatient care received a follow-up mental health visit within 7 days (Fontanella et al., 2015). In addition, non-Hispanic Black and other racially and ethnically diverse youth are less likely than non-Hispanic White youth to receive follow-up care from mental health care after psychiatric hospitalization (Merikangas et al., 2011). Moreover, context and settings are critical for youth populations, as racially and ethnically diverse youth are more likely to access mental health care services in school settings compared with community settings or community clinics (Cummings et al., 2010; Jaycox et al., 2010). This is particularly noteworthy in the context of the COVID-19 pandemic, said Barksdale, because these youth could not attend school in person and as a result have not been able to access their usual source of mental health care.

The reasons why racially and ethnically diverse groups may not be using or are underutilizing mental health services vary, but some of the most cited reasons include stigma surrounding seeking help (Eylem et al., 2020), structural inequalities in the mental health care service system (Nazroo et al., 2020; Williams, 2018), and limited knowledge of and access to resources (McGuire and Miranda, 2008). Other reasons include the limited availability of culturally and linguistically competent or culturally appropriate services and limited mental health literacy. For individuals living in rural areas, research suggests that individuals at elevated risk of suicide are less likely than those living in urban communities to have received mental health treatment (Cantrell et al., 2012; Fontanella et al., 2015), and they are more likely to use a firearm in suicide attempts (Searles et al., 2014). Barksdale said multiple factors contribute to rural populations underutilizing mental health services, including a shortage of mental health care providers, the lengthy distance to care providers, low mental health literacy, low perceived need, concerns about confidentiality, and stigma. Even when individuals living in rural areas do seek care, they do so later, often with more serious symptoms, and requiring more intensive treatments than their urban counterparts, said Barksdale.

Regarding mental health services use among sexual and gender minorities, research suggests that lesbian, gay, bisexual, transgender, queer and/or questioning, intersex, and asexual (LGBTQIA+) adults and youth, and particularly those who identify as transgender or gender diverse, are less likely to seek general community mental health services than non-LGBTQIA+ individuals (Craig et al., 2019) and they experience higher risk of suicide ideation (Oransky et al., 2019; Russon et al., 2021). Even when LGBTQIA+ individuals do access such services, they often report a high level of dissatisfaction with the services they receive. Transgender individuals, for example, have significantly different experiences in accessing care, specifically in terms of being denied care and experiencing discrimination. Reasons for underutilization by LGBTQIA+ individuals, said Barksdale, include a lack of family support and lack of support to seek services, concerns about privacy and disclosure, stigma, and a lack of available services that are affirming toward LGBTQIA+ individuals.

Turning to opportunities and next steps, Barksdale highlighted CDC's social-ecological model of suicide prevention that accounts for the complex interplay between individual, relationship, community, and societal factors.[5] This four-tier framework organizes risk and protective factors that can illustrate how one level might influence others and then inform corresponding multilevel intervention and prevention strategies that she believes are critical to addressing the complex issue of suicide prevention.

There are certainly opportunities to improve data collection, said Barksdale, particularly epidemiologic data on minoritized youth and intersectional populations. There are also opportunities to improve the ability to identify individuals, especially minoritized youth, who are at risk of completing a suicide attempt. In addition, more information and research are needed on the best approaches to prevent suicide, particularly among minoritized youth, and ensuring these approaches are both developmentally appropriate and culturally relevant. Barksdale concluded her remarks with a list of research opportunities available at NIMH detailed in Box 2.

---

[5] Additional information is available at https://www.cdc.gov/violenceprevention/about/social-ecologicalmodel.html (accessed October 25, 2021).

> **BOX 2**
> **Research Opportunities Available at NIMH**
>
> - Notice of Special Interest (NOSI) in Research on Risk and Prevention of Black Youth Suicide, https://grants.nih.gov/grants/guide/notice-files/NOT-MH-20-055
> - Systems-Level Risk Detection and Interventions to Reduce Suicide, Ideation, and Behaviors in Black Children and Adolescents (R01 Clinical Trial Optional), https://grants.nih.gov/grants/guide/rfa-files/RFA-MH-21-185.html
> - Systems-Level Risk Detection and Interventions to Reduce Suicide, Ideation, and Behaviors in Black Children and Adolescents (R34 Clinical Trial Optional), https://grants.nih.gov/grants/guide/rfa-files/RFA-MH-21-186.html
> - Systems-Level Risk Detection and Interventions to Reduce Suicide, Ideation, and Behaviors in Youth from Underserved Populations (R01 Clinical Trial Optional), https://grants.nih.gov/grants/guide/rfa-files/RFA-MH-21-187.html
> - Systems-Level Risk Detection and Interventions to Reduce Suicide, Ideation, and Behaviors in Youth from Underserved Populations (R34 Clinical Trial Optional), https://grants.nih.gov/grants/guide/rfa-files/RFA-MH-21-188.html
>
> SOURCE: Presented by Crystal L. Barksdale on June 22, 2021, at the workshop on Strategies and Interventions to Reduce Suicide.

OPPORTUNITIES IN HEALTH CARE TO REDUCE SUICIDE RISK

Following the two presentations, Holly C. Wilcox, professor at the Johns Hopkins Bloomberg School of Public Health, and Richard McKeon, chief of the Suicide Prevention Branch at the Substance Abuse and Mental Health Services Administration (SAMHSA), joined Bridge and Barksdale to answer questions from the workshop participants and to offer a few comments of their own. Jane Pearson, special advisor to the director on suicide research at NIMH, served as the discussion moderator.

Wilcox emphasized the pressing need to have layered suicide prevention approaches that include policies and protocols for workflow; training; developmentally timed, layered, evidence-based practices; coordination across systems of care; and better use of data for action. She also reiterated Barksdale's point that there are many barriers to engaging youth and adults in the traditional array of mental health services. "We lose people along each link in the chain of care," said Wilcox, who noted that there is some promise in leveraging technology to overcome some of those barriers to care. Wilcox also highlighted the importance of focusing more effort upstream to prevent crises from happening in the first place.

McKeon raised the issue that the Garrett Lee Smith Campus Suicide Prevention Grant Program,[6] which SAMHSA funds, is limited by law to the 10–24 age group. This is unfortunate, he said, because research has shown there is a sustained effect after consecutive years of programming, so starting that programming at a younger age might lead to an even larger positive effect on suicide rates in future years. The other implication of that finding is that suicide prevention programming cannot be "one and done." He also noted that the impact of Garrett Lee Smith grants was greater in rural communities than in other communities, though not in frontier communities (Walrath et al., 2015).

The second point McKeon made was that people at risk for suicide who have made suicide attempts are not getting the mental health care they need. "We have to be aware that there are many people at risk who are just not getting into our care systems, and we need to be able to pay better attention to them," said McKeon.

The first question for the panelists asked about when data from 2020 will be available. Bridge replied that national mortality data are available about 1 year later, so 2020 data should be available around December 2021. Bridge also noted that CDC has developed a system that provides provisional mortality estimates on a quarterly basis, which does allow for rapid surveillance of the issues.

In response to a question about the role of religious culture and suicide, Pearson asked Barksdale to comment on the religious settings in which some subgroups would potentially feel more or less comfortable. Barksdale replied that there have been several studies that included religion and religious settings as a source of care, which have shown that some individuals prefer to seek help from their religious care provider or their source of religion and have done so quite well (Harris et al., 2021; Hays and Lincoln, 2017), while other individuals have seen that as a source of stigma (Misra et al., 2021). "I think it depends on the cultural relevance of the help-seeking source," said Barksdale. Understanding help-seeking preferences is important, and there has been work on that subject, as well as on engaging religious institutions around mental health and suicide prevention.

---

[6] See https://www.samhsa.gov/newsroom/press-announcements/202106251130 (accessed October 25, 2021).

Responding to a question about the role that schools can play in suicide prevention, Wilcox said that schools can be an important component of upstream interventions. "If we can reach youth early, well in advance of a small issue becoming a big problem, we will make tremendous strides in reducing suicidal behavior," she said. Schools, however, cannot do this alone, and care transitions are absolutely critical between settings that can screen for suicide risk and settings that can intervene. Having a defined pathway for referrals into treatment would make it easier for schools and other screening settings to be part of an integrated system of care.

When asked about the role the 9-1-1 emergency call system can play in suicide prevention, McKeon said the issue is whether suicidal thoughts should always be considered an immediate emergency, and whether the response to such an emergency would be to use whatever means possible to get someone to the emergency department. "There is reason to think that is not the most effective system," said McKeon McKeon, adding "To the extent to which we can make emergency departments less central as part of a comprehensive suicide prevention response, I think there are many significant advantages to that, simultaneous with trying to improve care in the emergency department and, very importantly, improve follow-up afterward."

Based on a cohort study, explained McKeon, research has shown that people who made suicide attempts and who were seen in the emergency department had a 56-fold higher rate of death by suicide over the next 12 months, compared to general population patients who also visited the emergency department in the same 1-year period (Goldman-Mellor et al., 2019).

EXPERIENCES IN IMPLEMENTING SUICIDE PREVENTION CARE IN FEDERAL HEALTH CARE SETTINGS

Assessment and Management of Those at Risk for Suicide

Lisa Brenner, professor at the University of Colorado School of Medicine and director of the U.S. Department of Veterans Affairs (VA) Rocky Mountain Mental Illness Research, Education, and Clinical Center (MIRECC), discussed clinical practice guidelines and the role they can play in suicide prevention. The VA issued its clinical practice guidelines in 2019[7] to incorporate the significant leap in knowledge that had taken place over the 6 years since the VA released its previous guidelines. The VA developed the guidelines through a process of assembling multidisciplinary experts who developed 12 key questions, having an independent third party conduct a systematic review

---

[7] See https://www.healthquality.va.gov/guidelines/MH/srb (accessed October 25, 2021).

of the evidence relevant to those questions, and using a model of that looks at population, intervention, comparison or control, outcome, and time period, known as the PICOTS framework (Riva et al., 2012), to develop 22 recommendations that would put the best evidence into clinical practice. She noted that in many cases, sufficient research has yet to be conducted, highlighting an opportunity to engage in continued rigorous efforts to evaluate practices as a means of augmenting the existing evidence base.

As an example, one question the experts posed aimed to identify the most effective treatment approaches for patients identified as being most at risk for attempting suicide, particularly with regard to who was at risk and where and when to deliver an intervention. Brenner noted that this question highlighted an important point, which is that most of the research relevant to this question did not include minority populations and thus the findings may not hold for individuals from different backgrounds, different sexual orientations, gender identities, and different histories.

Of the 22 recommendations, 5 pertain to screening and evaluation, 12 to risk management and treatment, and 5 to other care management modalities including population- and community-based interventions. Brenner noted that each recommendation has a "strength" notation that indicates how strong the evidence is in favor or against a specific clinical practice. As an example, she cited one of the screening and evaluation recommendations that states,

> We recommend an assessment of risk factors as part of a comprehensive evaluation of suicide risk, including but not limited to current suicidal ideation, prior suicide attempt(s), current psychiatric conditions (e.g., mood disorders, substance use disorders) or symptoms (e.g., hopelessness, insomnia, agitation), prior psychiatric hospitalization, recent biopsychosocial stressors, and the availability of firearms.

Brenner noted that the evidence is strong for this recommendation. She added that in many cases, these recommendations line up with requirements for accrediting bodies.

The risk management and treatment recommendations include four pertaining to nonpharmacologic treatment, three to pharmacologic treatment and post-acute care, and two to technology-based treatment modalities. Brenner also noted that nonpharmacologic interventions include one for which the evidence is strong—using interventions based on cognitive behavioral therapy that are focused on suicide prevention for patients with a recent history of self-directed violence to reduce incidents of future self-directed violence—and three for which the supporting evidence is weak—offering dialectical behavioral therapy to individuals with borderline personality disorder and recent self-directed violence; offering psychotherapies based on problem solving to three specific groups of patients, and completing a crisis response plan for individuals with suicidal ideation or a lifetime history of suicide attempts. While the evidence supporting the use of these plans is weak, the VA highly recommends that clinicians engage in this type of activity, which is also an accreditation requirement. Brenner said that the VA clinical practice guideline website contains a variety of resources for each recommendation, as well as three clinical algorithms for clinicians.[8]

PROMOTING LETHAL MEANS SAFETY AMONG VETERANS: OPPORTUNITIES AND CHALLENGES

Lethal means safety is an intentional, voluntary practice to reduce access to lethal methods of suicide in order to reduce suicide risk, explained Joseph Simonetti, a physician and suicide prevention researcher at the VA Rocky Mountain MIRECC. This can be accomplished using a cable lock to secure a firearm, storing a firearm or ammunition outside of the home, or keeping medications in a secure lockbox stored away from those in a household who are at risk of suicide. Reduced access to lethal methods is one of the evidence-based methods for reducing suicide rates at the population level, said Simonetti. For that reason, the VA clinical practice guidelines, as well as various medical and public health professional societies, promote lethal means safety counseling or firearm safety counseling for individuals with elevated suicide risk. He added that in the VA, discussing how to reduce access to firearms is a key focus of lethal means safety counseling because 70 percent of veterans who die by suicide do so with a firearm (see Figure 10).

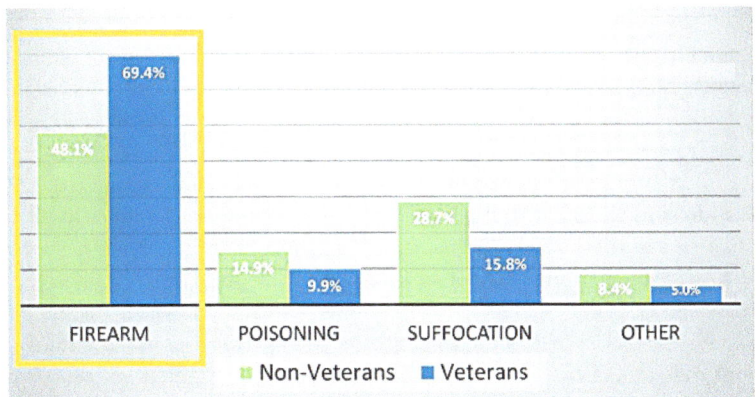

FIGURE 10 The role of firearms and other lethal means in suicides for veterans and nonveterans.
SOURCE: Presented by Joseph Simonetti on June 22, 2021, at the workshop on Strategies and Interventions to Reduce Suicide; VA, 2019.

---

[8] Additional information is available at https://www.healthquality.va.gov/guidelines/MH/srb (accessed October 25, 2021).

In practice, VA clinicians provide lethal means safety counseling as part of a safety plan, which is developed for patients with identified suicide risk. In addition, the VA now has an effort under way to provide standalone firearm safety counseling for patients with other identified injury risk factors. Simonetti explained that the VA is now supporting clinicians in providing firearm safety counseling across a wide array of clinical settings and different scenarios, and it has begun developing training resources for individuals in the firearm retail industry to parallel the VA's counseling efforts. At the same time, he added, the VA's research portfolio related to firearm injury prevention in general and suicide prevention specifically has expanded to ensure the VA is delivering high-quality and evidence-based interventions to its at-risk patients.

Simonetti suggested that one reason the VA has been able to establish itself as a leader in this field is its preexisting infrastructure and expertise in suicide prevention that is centrally coordinated. "That means we are able to rapidly disseminate resources to the field and reach a broad number of clinicians, and thus a large number of patients, through most of our efforts," said Simonetti. Another reason why the VA has been able to move forward with this effort is that there is a high level of acceptability throughout the VA system for having these types of conversations in clinical spaces. For example, the 2019 National Firearms Survey (Simonetti et al., 2021) shows that between 80 and 90 percent of those who live in U.S. households with firearms agree that clinicians should initiate firearm safety discussions when someone is at risk of suicide. In addition, there is widespread recognition that veterans are at elevated risk of suicide (Nelson et al., 2017). During a 2021 interview, when asked about discussing firearm safety with clinicians, one veteran told Simonetti that it was not bothersome that information came from clinicians because he trusts them, and while it seemed that this was nobody's business but his, he recognized that too many veterans are dying by suicide and so this went beyond his personal beliefs (Newell et al., 2021).

That being said, Simonetti noted there are a few important challenges to address to realize the full potential of lethal means safety counseling. First, lethal means safety counseling is not a single intervention; rather, it needs to be provided across many different settings and through different messengers delivering different messages to a heterogeneous mix of at-risk populations. In addition, researchers are challenged to develop and disseminate interventions that are effective, feasible, and tailored to these different audiences and settings.

Another challenge, he noted, is related to efforts to move suicide prevention interventions upstream. "This is critical because we know that many of our patients who go on to die by suicide are not engaged in specialty mental health treatment or safety planning," he said. Moving upstream by shifting the responsibilities for these tasks to clinical spaces that may be less accustomed to mental health treatment or suicide prevention generally is likely to require a shift in clinical practice for many clinicians and perhaps even a shift in clinical culture. "It is one thing to provide a psychologist with better tools to deliver firearm safety counseling," Simonetti, continuing,

> It may be a whole different challenge to begin thinking about how we facilitate the delivery of these discussions in medical and surgical subspecialty settings, for example, that do not consider suicide prevention within their clinical purview or wheelhouse.

Moving upstream will also require evidence that these interventions will remain acceptable and effective in the upstream setting. Simonetti notes that one thing that research has made clear is that while in general there is a high level of acceptability in terms of discussing lethal means safety, clinical context matters (Dobscha et al., 2021; Richards et al., 2021; Simonetti et al., 2020). Simply put, patients want to know why they are being asked about their firearms, said Simonetti.

In his final remarks, he noted that media reporting has suggested that firearm sales have surged, marked by purchases from different demographic groups and those who have different ownership motives, including individuals who have a wide range of prior training and experience with respect to firearm safety. The result, said Simonetti, is that these new gun purchasers may also have different firearm safety behaviors (Lyons et al., 2021). One study even found that individuals who purchased firearms for the first time during the COVID-19 pandemic were more likely to have suicidal ideation than other firearm owners (Anestis et al., 2021). "It is unclear whether the past year has spawned these unique risk populations that we know very little about in terms of both their suicide risk and their firearm safety behaviors," he said. Indeed, he added, much of the research in the qualitative and survey literature has focused on understanding the perspectives of the population that is familiar with firearms and how that population tends to have different perspectives and experiences from those that do not own or experience firearms regularly.

What is needed, he said, is research to understand the perspectives of people who own and/or live with firearms based on other characteristics such as gender or experiences with racial discrimination or trauma. Otherwise, said Simonetti, public health will continue to be at a disadvantage in trying to explain why suicide risk and rates may differ and be on different trajectories among specific populations. "That limits our ability to think about how we should be tailoring our approaches," he noted in closing. "This is work we desperately need to pursue if we are going to develop and eventually disseminate patient-centered interventions related to firearm safety and lethal means safety."

SUICIDE PREVENTION AND CARE PROGRAM

Pamela End of Horn, the national suicide prevention consultant to the Indian Health Service's (IHS's) Office of Clinical and Preventive Services, discussed IHS's efforts to work with national and local tribal communities on suicide prevention. Suicide, she noted, is a significant issue to Indian country—suicide is the eighth leading cause of death among all American Indian and Alaska Native communities across all ages—and it is one that can take over entire communities. The Suicide Prevention and Care program, she explained, operates in conjunction with programs in mental health and substance use disorders and with the IHS Telebehavioral Health Center of Excellence[9] to provide programs to tribal communities and tribal nations that focus on behavioral health care and suicide prevention.[10]

IHS, explained End of Horn, is a health care system, but, unlike the VA, it is more of a set of systems than one system in that it has federal partners, tribal partners, and local partners. Noting that the focus of IHS is on upstream models of care, she explained:

> We work to empower local tribal communities to take what we can provide them in regard to program offering, funding, information, evidence-based practices, best practice models, and help them implement them at the local level.

Regarding suicide prevention and care, she and her colleagues are engaged in the Ask Suicide-Screening Questions (ASQ) Toolkit pilot project (Horowitz et al., 2013; LeCloux et al., 2020), the IHS Substance Abuse Suicide Prevention Program,[11] and the Zero Suicide Initiative (Layman et al., 2021; Stapelberg et al., 2021), as well as developing the IHS community crisis response guidelines for addressing suicide behavior-related crises.[12]

The Zero Suicide model, explained End of Horn, is a comprehensive approach to suicide care that aims to reduce the risk of suicide for all individuals seen in health care systems (detailed in Box 3). Zero Suicide represents a bold commitment to patient safety, she said, holds the belief that the entire health system has the responsibility for preventing suicide deaths for patients under care. Zero Suicide promotes the use of seven elements to improve patient safety—lead, train, identify, engage, treat, transition, and improve—as being essential to improving patient safety. She noted that most of the Zero Suicide pilot sites are located in the U.S. Southwest, with three in Navajo

---

[9] See https://www.ihs.gov/telebehavioral (accessed October 25, 2021).
[10] See https://www.ihs.gov/telebehavioral (accessed October 25, 2021).
[11] See https://www.ihs.gov/sasp/aboutsasp (accessed October 25, 2021).
[12] See https://www.ihs.gov/suicideprevention/communityguidelines (accessed October 25, 2021).

> **BOX 3**
> **Key Features of the Zero Suicide Initiative**
>
> - Documentation of ideation with plan, attempts, and completions among all patients
> - A comprehensive, system-wide suicide care policy that addresses screening, assessment, safety planning, treatment, and follow up
> - A quality assurance process that monitors adherence to suicide care policy and clinical protocols on all levels
> - Universal screening for suicide risk in the health system
> - Full suicide risk assessments for all patients that screen positive for suicide risk
> - Collaboratively developed safety plans completed for all patients at moderate to high risk for suicide
> - Timely follow up for all patients during care transitions
> - Establishing an electronic health record that facilitates tracking of at-risk patients and delvers timely, relevant data
> - Use of culturally informed and traditional practices with evidence-based practices
>
> SOURCE: Presented by Pamela End of Horn on June 22, 2021, at the workshop on Strategies and Interventions to Reduce Suicide.

areas, one each in Phoenix, Albuquerque, and Oklahoma City, as well as two in the north in Bemidji, Minnesota, and Billings, Montana. This wide swath of sites requires adapting how the model is implemented to reflect local cultures.

The pilot program, said End of Horn, established cooperative agreements with the tribal governments so that she and her colleagues could work closely with the tribes to understand how best to apply the model, how it works in different cultures, and what the tribes needed to do within their health systems to improve care and prevent suicides. The pilot program ended in 2021. She noted that while the COVID-19 pandemic created significant challenges to the program, particularly with regard to in-person to health care facilities, it also made the tribes realize that they can implement this type of model within the community and within their schools. One site, for example, established a COVID-19 hotline that people could call if they were feeling overwhelmed or suicidal and needed to gain access to resources. "It helped the community find a cohesive response to the issue of the pandemic and the reality that they were facing in regard to what was happening at the local level," she said. The new perspective that the local sites have gained from the COVID-19 pandemic is something that she hopes to maintain.

The pilot program has also encountered a number of challenges, including high staff turnover and having to invest in retraining, as well as the need to have staff dedicated to case management and follow up. Other challenges have included establishing and maintaining participation with primary care, a lack of collaboration with community health facilities following inpatient discharge, a lack of data-sharing agreements that hinders assessment and continuous improvement activities, and the difficulty of retrofitting electronic health records (EHRs) to embed screening, assessment, and tracking tools.

Going forward, said End of Horn, she and her colleagues plan to use crisis lines to assist with follow-up contacts and use case managers to conduct continual tracking of patients in care pathways. They also plan to improve EHR functionality by adding alerts and establishing data-sharing agreements.

IMPROVING SUICIDE PREVENTION: ADDRESSING KNOWN BARRIERS TO HEALTH CARE ACCESS

Ursula Whiteside, chief executive officer at NowMattersNow.org and clinical faculty member at the University of Washington, introduced the next session by referring participants to the 2018 report from the National Action Alliance for Suicide Prevention, *Recommended Standard Care for People with Suicide Risk*,[13] which aims to help health systems better identify and support people who are at increased risk of suicide. In particular, she said, the report addresses some of the barriers that people at risk of suicide face in accessing care. "People with lived experience have all sorts of reasons for not reaching out for care or for having poor experiences when they do," she said.

Whiteside referred to a treatment called dialectical behavior therapy,[14] a form of cognitive behavior therapy that her team uses to understand the history and biology that informs where people are on a day-to-day level in terms of their stress. On a given day, for example, some people are more emotionally reactive than others based on different adverse life experiences, such as trauma or systemic injustice. "We think about this as being on fire emotionally, and the adverse experience may explain why people do things that they would not necessarily do otherwise" said Whiteside. She asked the workshop participants to consider this model (see Figure 11) of emotional dysregulation when thinking about a person during a crisis, adding that this model can also help family members and friends have a better understanding of what someone at risk of suicide may be experiencing.

Language matters, emphasized Whiteside. Based on feedback received from those who have had a personal experience related to suicide, health care

---

[13] The report is available for free at https://theactionalliance.org/sites/default/files/action_alliance_recommended_standard_care_final.pdf (accessed October 26, 2021).

[14] Additional information is available at https://behavioraltech.org/resources/faqs/dialectical-behavior-therapy-dbt (accessed October 26, 2021).

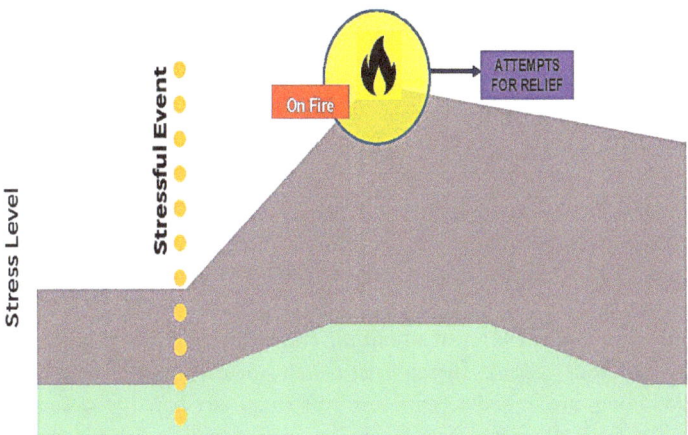

FIGURE 11 Emotional dysregulation can affect some people more than others when they respond to a stressful event.
SOURCE: Presented and created by Ursula Whiteside on June 22, 2021, at the workshop on Strategies and Interventions to Reduce Suicide.

providers and others should choose compassionate and accurate language when discussing suicide. Language should shift from using the term "committed suicide" to "died by suicide or died of suicide," and from "dealing with" suicidal patients to "working with" them. Similarly, she said, it is important to be thoughtful in describing behavior and not adding an interpretation, which means eliminating the use of phrases such as "manipulative," "attention seeking," "suicidal gesture," and "cry for help."

Whiteside noted that in the work she does, she is guided by a team of people with lived experience. The biggest take-home message they have is that all the interventions in the world may not help if the health care provider panics, does not show that they are with the individual in that moment of crisis, and cannot figure out a way to offer hope. "This is not in an 'It is going to be okay, I have all the answers' manner, but in a way that conveys they will help that person in crisis get through the next 5 minutes."

IMPROVING SUICIDE PREVENTION: ADDRESSING KNOWN BARRIERS TO HEALTH CARE ACCESS FOR LGBTQIA+ PEOPLE IN INSTITUTIONAL SETTINGS

With almost 2.1 million people, New Mexico is a culturally rich, mostly rural, economically challenged majority-minority state, explained Cathleen Willging, center director and senior research scientist at the Pacific Institute for Research and Evaluation's Southwest Center. Suicide is a leading cause of death, she continued, with the state experiencing higher rates of suicide than the U.S. average for the last quarter of the century. Rates of suicidal behaviors for LGBTQIA+ adults and youth far exceed those for heterosexual and cisgender New Mexicans (Whiteside, 2019; Whiteside and Green, 2021).

In 2019, more than 19 percent of sexual minority adults and 22 percent of gender minority adults in New Mexico had reportedly considered attempting to die by suicide (Personal communication from C. Whiteside to C. Willging, 2021), while 40 percent of LGBTQIA+ high school students had considered attempting to die by suicide, 34 percent developed a plan to do so, and 25 percent making an attempt in the past year (Ivey-Stephenson et al., 2020; Whiteside, 2019). These disparities in suicidal thoughts and behaviors, said Willging, are linked to exposure to structurally based stressors, such as discrimination, associated with being part of a socially stigmatized group, as opposed to being LGBTQIA+ in and of itself.

Willging noted that New Mexico is underserved medically, with most services concentrated in Albuquerque, while all or parts of 33 counties, accounting for 50 percent of the state's population, are designated primary care and health professional shortage areas (Avery et al., 2018). Some 60 percent of the state's residents live in mental health professional shortage areas, and in addition, the state's behavioral health system is fragmented and fragile, a situation exacerbated by the forced closure of community mental health centers in 2013 that created mental health care deserts throughout the state (Willging and Trott, 2018). This closure was caused by a political controversy that resulted in the New Mexico's Department of Health and Human Services removing Medicaid payments to 15 mental health providers after an audit reported credible evidence of fraud (Terrell, 2019). As a result, primary care clinics in the state are struggling to increase their service delivery capacity because there are few places to which they can refer patients, and appointments and waiting lists for services are long throughout the state of New Mexico. Furthermore, most practices have yet to try tailoring services to LGBTQIA+ patients.

Schools are another de facto source of support, Willging added, though there are less than 80 school-based health centers for New Mexico's 89 school districts and 867 schools (LESC, 2021a,b; LFC, 2021). Of the 89 school districts, 18 have less than one full-time school nurse, with more than one-third of the school-based nurses serving multiple campuses (Shattuck et al., 2021). In 2009, said Willging, 40 percent of the state's high school-based nurses provided emergency management for a suicidal student, a figure that increased to 75 percent in 2019 (Ramos et al., 2013; Shattuck et al., 2021).

Willging explained that her remarks draw from two studies shaped by implementation science.[15] The first study was a randomized cluster trial initiated in 2016 that used implementation science to enable the uptake of evidence-informed practices to make high schools safer and more supportive of LGBTQIA+ students, thereby reducing their risk for suicidal behavior (Green et al., 2018; Shattuck et al., 2020; Willging et al., 2016).[16] The second study used a mixed method research design to assess factors affecting access to quality primary care for LGBTQIA+ patients, focusing on clinical preparedness, implementation climates, and readiness for LGBTQIA+-centered care in clinical settings (Willging et al., 2020).[17]

Social institutions such as health systems and schools perpetuate cultural values of heteronormativity and cisgenderism that can harm the health of LGBTQIA+ people from youth into adulthood, said Willging, "the attitudes, language, and behaviors of health and school professionals can engender hostile climates, marginalizing LGBTQIA+ people and making them feel disconnected." Experiences of discrimination in these settings, such as the biased enforcement of rules that disproportionately target LGBTQIA+ youth and students of color, combined with the social pressures of being part of a minoritized group, contribute to school pushout and a domino effect of other negative consequences that can heighten a young person's risk for suicide as they age, she explained. Furthermore, when LGBTQIA+ people experience discrimination in health care settings, they may delay or avoid getting the care they need.

Willging noted that staff in health systems and schools commonly state that they treat everyone the same to signify that they do not discriminate, yet such attitudes may reduce the motivation to educate themselves and support evidence-informed policies and practices that might benefit the physical and mental health of LGBTQIA+ people. In addition, a pervasive lack of education among health and school professionals contributes to the invisibility of LGBTQIA+ people in institutional settings and low awareness of their unique mental health needs.

Several barriers thwart access to needed supports in schools, said Willging. To start, the paucity of school-based health care professionals creates hardships

---

[15] Implementation science is the scientific study of methods and strategies that facilitate the uptake of evidence-based practice and research into regular use by practitioners and policymakers. More information can be found at https://impsciuw.org/implementation-science/learn/implementation-science-overview (accessed November 29, 2021).

[16] Additional information is available at https://southwest.pire.org/project/implementing-school-nursing-strategies-to-reduce-lgbtq-adolescent-suicide (accessed October 26, 2021).

[17] Additional information is available at https://southwest.pire.org/project/enhancing-primary-care-services-for-diverse-sexual-and-gender-minority-populations (accessed October 26, 2021).

in identifying or responding to any student with suicidal behaviors. Moreover, school staff are often unsure as to whether community-based care providers are LGBTQIA+ competent or accepting. In addition, the professional development of school staff on suicide prevention and intervention occurs infrequently, is seldom reinforced through follow-up training, and typically is not a priority for school leadership unless it is student or community initiated. She added that because of high turnover rates across schools, many staff are unlikely to receive even basic training to address suicide.

Willging et al. (2016) has found that school staff often cite low mental health literacy and insufficient engagement among parents and guardians as major challenges in making sure students experiencing suicidal behaviors get support. In addition, stigma about having their children identified as having mental health concerns or as queer creates further resistance among parents to seek needed services and support. In the same way, primary care providers point to the difficulties of delivering private, confidential care to at-risk LGBTQIA+ youth without accepting families.

In addition to the challenges of accessing needed services in schools, Willging said there are additional barriers to addressing the needs of LGBTQIA+ people at risk for suicide. The primary care providers and staff she and her colleagues have talked to make it clear that clinics could be doing more to engage in outreach and to advertise their services to LGBTQIA+ people to pull patients in for care. They report not knowing much about LGBTQIA+ resources outside their clinics, including where to get training or where to refer patients with mental health concerns, such as LGBTQIA+ support groups. One reason outreach is not happening, she noted, is that administrators are not seeing a need to engage in those types of activities. "LGBTQIA+ people remain off the radar, and the demand for LGBTQIA+-responsive services is deemed low," said Willging. "Not having electronic medical records setup to collect and use data on the gender identities and sexual orientations of patients, or staff prepared to ask appropriate questions to get this information, likely contributes to perceptions of low demand."

Worse yet, during Willging's research, she found that administrators in some places do not want to create LGBTQIA+-responsive services because they do not want to make non-LGBTQIA+ patients resentful or uncomfortable. Having to care for patients of varying ages and cultural backgrounds also makes it hard to justify innovating services for LGBTQIA+ people, said Willging. This contributes to the siloing of expertise in which only a minority of staff may possess the knowledge and skills necessary to work with LGBTQIA+ patients, particularly with respect to gender affirming care.

One major finding from her two studies is that people do not know what they do not know. "Until they started taking part in our studies, many folks we talked to had not given much attention to LGBTQIA+ issues in their workplace, so they did not have a reason to prioritize or invest in inclusive services or supports," said Willging. "Because these issues are on the periphery of their radar screens, if at all, preparedness to intervene appropriately to reduce negative health and mental health outcomes for LGBTQIA+ people is minimal." On the other hand, her research showed that through professional development, it is possible to make substantial inroads toward enabling people working in these institutional settings to become more involved and to initiate the processes of organizational change.

In terms of what institutions can do to reduce access barriers and health disparities for LGBTQIA+ individuals, there are evidence-informed practices available. Schools, for example, can establish safe spaces and social groups on campus that promote school connectedness among LGBTQIA+ students, a major protective factor against suicidal behaviors. Schools can also adopt inclusive curricula that do not neglect LGBTQIA+ health concerns and that foster mental health literacy. They can also vet community health care providers and confirm they are knowledgeable about and provide supportive care for LGBTQIA+ people. In fact, she and her colleagues have collaborated with schools to organize LGBTQIA+ 101 trainings for local care providers, attracting them by offering free continuing education credits.

Primary care clinics can do more as well, particularly in terms of creating a welcoming environment. Steps they can take include increasing outreach efforts in the communities they serve, transitioning to gender-neutral restrooms, and displaying artwork and educational materials that signify their support. Clinics can also start collecting and using data on gender identity and sexual orientation as part of routine clinical care and make it possible for staff to understand and address disparities affecting LGBTQIA+ patients. In addition, primary care clinics have a responsibility to ensure, through targeted workforce development, that LGBTQIA+ patients receive care in keeping with national recommendations and best practices.

Willging said that everyone working in schools and primary care should be expected to—and empowered to—become familiar with basic approaches to cultural competency when interacting with LGBTQIA+ people. They also need to be proficient in using common LGBTQIA+ terminology, as well as supporting and enforcing antidiscrimination policies as a means of guarding against marginalizing LGBTQIA+ people. Finally, she added, by forging connections with LGBTQIA+ communities, such as with advocacy organizations, schools and clinics will find eager collaborators willing to make these things possible.

There are, however, social factors, pragmatic considerations, and leadership issues that can get in the way of introducing innovations that support populations such as LGBTQIA+ people that experience health disparities and increased risk for suicide. For example, being from a small socially conservative community where stigma surrounding mental health and LGBTQIA+ issues abounds can make staff less likely to get visibly engaged as change champions. Time constraints, being overworked, and lack of resources can also get in the way of implementing LGBTQIA+-inclusive practices in schools and clinics. So, too, can misalignment among different leaders within an organization. In one case, Willging shared, school nurse leaders were eagerly awaiting the receipt of implementation support for suicide prevention, but their principals unilaterally withdrew from Willging's school study based on their personal beliefs that LGBTQIA+ students did not warrant special intervention. Leaders may also deprioritize LGBTQIA+-directed initiatives for less problematic reasons, as their time and energy are often devoted to ensuring that schools and clinics comply with the many state and federal mandates governing education and health care delivery.

While institutions need to change and foster suicide prevention and intervention for populations with health disparities, Willging said that society cannot demand change without investing in the institutions and people who work within them to do things differently. Professional development that cultivates knowledge and reflection on the social causes of ill health and understanding of the reasons behind inadequate or fragmented support is critical, she said, adding that it cannot be done in a single training. Willging briefly noted that while focusing on health risk behaviors at the individual level is useful for professional development, it can also reinforce stigma and stereotypes when it is not paired with attention to structural and systemic processes that exacerbate inequities for minoritized social groups. In that respect, adopting a structural competency framework to organize professional development can be useful by enhancing awareness of upstream factors such as stigma and discrimination that abet marginalization and give way to disproportionate risks for suicidal behaviors. Such a framework can also enhance the case for larger-order, focused interventions directed at changing implementation environments, overcoming institutional inertia, and doing something about adverse health outcomes for particular social groups.

Making a pitch for using implementation science to overcome barriers, Willging said there are conceptual frameworks to guide change processes and promote access to suicide prevention and intervention in institutional settings. Two frameworks she mentioned were the Consolidated Framework for Implementation Research (Damschroder et al., 2009) and the Exploration, Preparation, Implementation, and Sustainment framework (Aarons et al., 2011). These frameworks focus on multiple stages and levels of influence during change processes, encouraging initial and ongoing assessment of factors at the outer context, including the broader system environment, policy, funding, and community stigma, as well as inner context factors, or characteristics internal to a school or clinic, such as staff and leader attitudes and behaviors. They also offer roadmaps for crafting climates conducive to successful implementation.

Implementation science also offers tools to increase the uptake of new programs or practices. Two strategies for promoting stakeholder engagement and building capacity among diverse stakeholders to wrestle with health disparities include the dynamic adaptation process (Aarons et al., 2012) and implementation facilitation (Ritchie et al., 2020). As a final comment, Willging said that implementation science is about addressing messy but important problems, including health disparities and structural incompetence. She said,

> Addressing such problems is complex and takes time, but [it] is essential to carrying out evidence-based suicide prevention and intervention in schools, clinics, and other institutional settings, and for reducing high rates of suicidal behaviors for health disparity populations.

RISK ID: THE VA SUICIDE RISK IDENTIFICATION STRATEGY

One way to improve the availability of suicide prevention services is by upstream screening and evaluation, which the VA has been striving to implement throughout its health care system, not just in mental health specialty care, said Brenner. The VA's Suicide Risk Identification Strategy program (Risk ID) is a national, standardized process for suicide risk screening and evaluation using high-quality, evidence-based tools and practices to facilitate and encourage fidelity to best screening and evaluation practices. "This is the largest effort that has been undertaken in any health care system in the United States," she said, adding that the VA has screened about 6 million people using Risk ID, including many who would not have been seen in a specialty clinic.

Risk ID outlines a clear process for who should be screened and evaluated, when screening or evaluation should occur, and how screening or evaluation should be conducted and documented. It includes a universal requirement that every veteran will be screened by an appropriate staff member. Specific clinical settings in which the veteran is known to be at risk have additional screening and evaluation requirements (see Table 1), said Brenner, who added that Risk ID is also indicated when a new behavioral health concern is evident. By including these different clinical settings, the VA now has many more health care providers who understand that suicide prevention is part of their daily business and that they are responsible for it in their screening and treatment situations. She also noted that the process of screening and evaluation has evolved over time with new evidence and that the VA expects it will continue to evolve as the program continues to gather data.

The two-step Risk ID process uses the Columbia-Suicide Severity Rating Scale (C-SSRS), a validated, evidence-supported questionnaire available in 103

TABLE 1 Minimum Screening Requirements by Setting for Risk ID

Setting	Requirements (in addition to Annual Screening)
Emergency Department and Urgent Care Centers	C-SSRS Screener at each encounter (is embedded in the National Emergency Department/Urgent Care RN Triage note)
Outpatient Mental Health	C-SSRS Screener during intake evaluation; as clinically indicated thereafter
Sleep Clinic	C-SSRS Screener at referral or intake; C-SSRS Screener must be completed during intake evaluation if > 30 days from referral; as clinically indicated thereafter
Pain Clinic	C-SSRS Screener at referral or intake; C-SSRS Screener must be completed during intake evaluation if > 30 days from referral; as clinically indicated thereafter
Opioid Treatment Program	C-SSRS Screener during intake evaluation; as clinically indicated thereafter. In cases of administrative discharge, CSRE within 24 hours before discharge if the patient can be reached.
Mental Health Residential Rehabilitation Treatment Program	C-SSRS Screener within 24 hours of admission and CSRE during the first week of admission; updated CSRE within a week before discharge and C-SSRS within 24 hours before discharge
Community Living Center	C-SSRS Screener within 24 hours of admission and within 24 hours before discharge
Inpatient Mental Health	C-SSRS Screener within 24 hours of admission and within 24 hours before discharge
Inpatient Medical/Surgical	C-SSRS Screener within 24 hours of admission and within 24 hours before discharge
Inpatient & Residential Rehabilitation	C-SSRS Screener within 24 hours of admission and within 24 hours before discharge

NOTE: C-SSRS = Columbia-Suicide Severity Rating Scale; CSRE = VA Comprehensive Suicide Risk Evaluation.
SOURCE: Presented by Lisa Brenner on June 22, 2021, at the workshop on Strategies and Interventions to Reduce Suicide.

different languages.[18] A positive C-SSRS score requires the timely completion of the VA Comprehensive Suicide Risk Evaluation (CSRE), which would be on the same day in the ambulatory care setting and with 24 hours in inpatient or residential settings. The CSRE is designed to inform clinical impressions about acute and chronic risk and associated disposition, thereby allowing clinicians to match the risk level with an appropriate treatment.

To support staff that may not be accustomed to conducting suicide risk screening, VA has developed a number of additional trainings, laminated

---

[18] The C-SSRS questionnaire and additional information is available at https://suicide preventionlifeline.org/wp-content/uploads/2016/09/Suicide-Risk-Assessment-C-SSRS-Lifeline-Version-2014.pdf (accessed November 5, 2021).

screening materials, and dashboards that clinicians can review to see how well they are doing. Risk ID includes a technical support email address and call center as well. "We are trying to support care providers in different settings and in different types of care and implement this as a whole-of-enterprise process," said Brenner. The dashboard, for example, helps clinicians identify who they are missing and why, which not only helps improve overall levels of practice, but also provides information on workflows and practice settings that can help local clinics improve their operations.

One of the initial assessments of Risk ID demonstrated that instituting a universal screening plan is possible with commitment and technical assistance (Bahraini et al., 2020). This study also showed that the risk level of veterans seen in the emergency department was higher than for those seen in an ambulatory care setting, which was not unexpected, said Brenner. The VA has begun collecting initial data regarding race, ethnicity, and other factors that should help the VA ensure that individuals from different backgrounds are receiving screening and evaluation though missing data limits the VA's ability to assess for health disparities by race (GAO, 2019).

Brenner's hope is that the VA will implement more evidence-based practices, conduct more systematic screening, and generate more data that will enable the system to do a better job of meeting the needs of all veterans equitably. As a closing comment, she said that the VA has a free consultation service available for clinicians treating veterans in community care settings.[19]

SUICIDE PREVENTION: BARRIERS TO CARE AMONG BLACK YOUTH AND FAMILIES

Between 1991 and 2017, 18.8 percent of U.S. high school–aged youth thought about suicide and 14.7 percent had formed a suicide plan (Lindsey et al., 2019), said Michael Lindsey, executive director of New York University's McSilver Institute for Poverty Policy and Research. Over the same period, he noted, suicide attempts for Black youth rose by 73 percent while falling for every other racial and ethnic group. Similarly, the rate of injury related to a suicide attempt for Black youth increased by 120 percent over that time. These increases occurred even while thinking about and planning suicide had actually decreased among Black youth over that period, which led Lindsey to wonder if Black youth might be going straight to a suicide attempt.

To explore that possibility, Lindsey and his collaborators used an ideation to action framework (Klonsky and May, 2015) to look at whether there are

---

[19] See https://www.ptsd.va.gov/professional/consult/index.asp (accessed October 26, 2021).

distinctions based on race in terms of which youth are engaging in different types of nonfatal suicide behaviors. He noted that many studies examine outcomes related to suicides by comparing youth who have engaged in suicide behavior compared to non-suicidal youth, whereas this study looks within the group of youth who have engaged in suicide behavior to see if there are any distinctions. The main finding from this study was that compared to youth of all other racial and ethnic groups, Black youth had higher odds of having an attempt only and no preceding thoughts or plans. "In terms of screening and prevention, this is scary when you think that the common warning signs we look for in terms of suicidal behavior might not be as apparent for Black youth," said Lindsey. In fact, he added, a recent study found that there is a higher rate of suicide misclassification for Black adolescents who died compared to their White counterparts (Ali et al., 2021).

Turning to the subject of barriers to care, Lindsey noted that large scale epidemiologic studies have shown that Black youth, relative to White youth, underuse specialty mental health care and receive less treatment for mood disorders (Costello et al., 2014). Research has also found that fewer than 50 percent of youth who access mental health treatment do so following an emergency department visit (Bridge et al., 2012; Rhodes et al., 2018).

In terms of barriers to care, Lindsey addressed two broad factors. Factor one, he said relates to the stigma associated with mental illness and service use and the primacy of family support. Qualitative studies he has conducted have found that Black youth prefer to take their problems, concerns, and cares to family members first, and in many cases, the family members then tell them not to take their problems outside of the family. Often, said Lindsey, Black youth who present with a mental health struggle are seen by their family members—and even educators—as simply being lazy, and therefore, are not likely to seek care for the child. In addition, there is a distrust of health care providers because of concern they will not understand a Black person's unique experiences and provide messages discordant with lived, contextual experiences or that the provider will misdiagnose or misclassify presenting symptoms.

The results of these attitudes are seen in a study Lindsey and his colleagues conducted in Baltimore. There, they found that about half of a sample of 465 ninth graders had identified mental health needs, but only 20 percent of those students received services, even when those services were available at their schools (Lindsey et al., 2010). All this, said Lindsey, argues for developing different types of interventions and strategies to employ when working with Black families, interventions that can overcome stigma and perceptual barriers to treatment. He noted that those Black youth who did access services reported that they had positive or supportive family networks.

The other broad factor that acts as a barrier to seeking care is the common misinterpretation of presenting symptoms in schools. For example it is well-established that youth with depression are likely to exhibit irritability, anger, and other kinds of negative behaviors as a manifestation of their depression. Lindsey said that because of implicit bias, a Black student exhibiting those behaviors is more likely to be suspended or expelled from school compared to a White student. In fact, Black students, boys, and children with disabilities are often overrepresented with regard to disproportionate discipline in school (GAO, 2018).

He noted another study showing that school children living in lower socioeconomic areas displayed the highest level of behavioral problems at the end of the month, which was associated with the family running out of Supplemental Nutrition Assistance Program benefits (Gennetian et al., 2016). The same group of investigators found that income instability also predicted student expulsions and suspensions (Gennetian et al., 2015). "Often, it seems to be the case that schools do not do that next level of inquiry about what kind of presenting issues or concerns that kid is bringing to the school, which in this instance is perhaps hunger," said Lindsey.

One important policy issue, Lindsey explained, has to do with the fact that fewer than 10 states across the nation require social and emotional learning standards from pre-kindergarten through 12th grade. Lindsey said,

> I think that it would be incredibly important for kids to understand how to process their emotions, how to reconcile interpersonal challenges that they have with others in a way that allows them to be able to understand their emotional processing, and then perhaps be at a place to ask for help as they need it.

The biggest policy action that could reduce or eliminate a barrier to care, he said, would be for every school to have available mental health care providers at a level proportionate to the number of children in a school. "What we find, particularly in communities of color, is that there is not a provider available at school, or if there is a provider, they are there only 1 day a week," he noted. This is why Lindsey and his colleagues, as well as members of Congress, have been advocating for the federal government to pay more attention to this issue (Coleman and Congressional Black Caucus, 2019) which led to the U.S. House of Representatives passing the Pursuing Equity in Mental Health Act in May 2021 by a margin of 349 to 74.

SUICIDE PREVENTION: STIGMA AND THE COVID-19 PANDEMIC

Session moderator Erin Bagalman, director of the Division of Behavioral Health Policy in the Office of the Assistant Secretary for Planning and Evaluation at the U.S. Department of Health and Human Services (HHS), opened the panel discussion by asking Willging to comment on suicide prevention in the context of the COVID-19 pandemic. Willging replied that she and her colleagues surveyed 379 self-identified LGBTQIA+ youth in New Mexico and found that during the pandemic 41 percent did not feel safe in the own homes because of their sexual orientations or gender expression.

In addition, over 83 percent felt sad or hopeless during the summer of 2020, 46 percent considered suicide during those early months of the pandemic, close to 33 percent made a plan for suicide, and 12 percent attempted suicide. She noted that during the pandemic, schools lost track of those kids who might be at risk, which left those youth without a de facto surveillance system. Limited broadband access in New Mexico has aggravated some of the mental health needs for these children and adolescents. "Even finding a private space to engage online with a mental health specialist was challenging for many youth, and we had several reports of youth telling us their parents were actively discouraging them from getting mental health support," said Willging. Another issue was that schools and teachers were so focused on making adjustments to conducting online instruction during the pandemic that suicide prevention and initiatives to support LGBTQIA+ youth were deprioritized.

Bagalman then asked End of Horn to comment on suicide prevention in the context of the racial tensions and civil unrest demonstrated in 2020 and 2021. End of Horn replied that the Black Lives Matter movement served as a wake-up call for many Native scholars to talk about how colonization, colonialism, and White supremacy have affect tribal nations, not only in terms of racial disparities but in terms of the high mortality and morbidity rates and the high rates of disease burdens. This awakening brought to the forefront the issue of how to contextualize suicide prevention without using colonial language to meet the unique needs of the Native population.

Simonetti noted that the pandemic, racial justice demonstrations, and other recent events have placed different stressors on different households, and people have interpreted these stressors in different ways. He said two primary concerns are the spike of firearm violence in many major cities in the country that has led to a "wholesale sense of urgency," and the increase in firearm purchases at a time when families have been clustered together under high-stress conditions. One question is whether this period will represent a short-lived change or if firearm ownership has changed for a large proportion of the country.

Brenner commented that she appreciated Lindsey noting that food insecurity and other factors not normally associated with suicide can, in fact, be suicide risk factors. Food insecurity and other financial challenges are risk factors for veterans, she noted, and the COVID-19 pandemic has introduced huge economic stresses into many families that have not experienced them before. It will be important, she said, to monitor how this confluence of stressors will play out over time. Lindsey agreed that it is time to consider some of the larger contextual factors and the role they play beyond traditional psychiatric symptoms in leading to engagement in suicidal behaviors.

Bagalman asked the panelists for their ideas on how to change the stigma, especially in the Black community, in order to address mental health as an illness rather than from a negative perspective. Lindsey replied with exemplar of a freestanding mental health clinic located in a church-associated facility that provides free services to all. As he noted, faith communities can play a critical role in combating stigma. Another opportunity is to revisit what is happening in schools with regard to so-called zero-tolerance policies and to instead provide the kinds of behavioral health supports that children need, including working with families to provide education about psychological issues. In fact, the whole idea of providing services in nontraditional settings can be used to combat stigma, he said.

Both Whiteside and Brenner commented on the importance of getting health care providers out of their offices to meet people where they are most comfortable receiving services, whether that be in their churches or at the firing range. Brenner noted the importance of getting unlikely partners to engage with the mental health community. Simonetti agreed and said that is happening in the firearm community. "Engaging those stakeholders provides a great opportunity for outreach and to build credibility in communities where we might not necessarily carry with us the most credibility," said Simonetti.

LEVELS OF PROGRESS TOWARD PREVENTION

Michael Hogan, principal at Hogan Health Solutions, concluded day one of the workshop with some of the key themes he observed throughout the day. "Suicide remains a major issue and despite some trends that may be positive … it remains a major issue and a major cause of unnecessary loss of life," says Hogan. But he also emphasized the progress that the VA has accomplished within its health care system, and he said it could serve as an example of what could be done in other health care contexts.

Hogan noted some positive changes in the expectations of accrediting organizations, including the Joint Commission and the Commission on Accreditation of Rehabilitation Facilities. However, he said it is time to provide consistent federal funding, such as a block grant rather than a competitive grant, for the Garrett Lee Smith Campus Suicide Prevention Grant Program.

When it comes to caring for people who are actively contemplating suicide, says Hogan, it is clear that connection and collaboration are crucial, that isolation is poisonous, and that directly dealing with thoughts and impulses from suicide is necessary and effective. "It is high time to bring those things, as we have in the VA, across the rest of our health care system," said Hogan. He noted that the nation is slowly beginning to evolve attitudes about race, and there is slow but remarkable progress with respect to attitudes about gender, and in understanding that both culture and gender are pivotal when it comes to suicidality.

Hogan concluded by saying that upstream suicide prevention efforts are important, but they are massively under-resourced. "We cannot pretend that we can achieve what needs to be done until we make a change," he said. The national movement to turn on 9-8-8 as a single emergency phone number next year for people in a mental health crisis can possibly be a turning point, "but it is only a beginning step and we have to do much more, especially upstream."

BUILDING 9-8-8: AN OPPORTUNITY TO BUILD INCLUSIVE CARE STRUCTURES

Through legislation, 9-8-8 has been designated the new nationwide emergency number to the National Suicide Prevention Lifeline.[20] By July 2022, Americans will be able to quickly connect with crisis counselors for easier access to life-saving resources. The second webinar of this workshop considered opportunities to build inclusive care and the implications of the 9-8-8 expansion initiative including the gaps, challenges, and needs for marginalized and vulnerable populations.

Mary Roary, director of the Office of Behavioral Health Equity at SAMHSA, opened the day by acknowledging that every 40 seconds, someone dies by suicide. After 40 seconds of silence in memory of those who have died by suicide, she reiterated the key themes that emerged during the first webinar on June 22, 2021, which were the importance of cultural competency, health equity, and addressing the barriers to suicide prevention, such as the lack of access to health care services and health care provider shortages, that are exacerbated by COVID-19 and the ongoing civil unrest. Roary noted that sustainability needs to be built into planning for suicide prevention programs and that there is a need for an extended research focus that targets traditionally under-resourced and marginalized groups such as American Indians and Alaska Natives, members of the LGBTQIA+ community, Black youth, military veterans, and people who are homeless.

IMPROVING CARE COORDINATION WITHIN CRISIS SERVICES

Mary Ann Nihart, associate director of patient care services and nurse executive for the San Francisco Veterans Affairs Healthcare System, recounted

---

[20] See https://www.congress.gov/bill/116th-congress/senate-bill/2661/all-info (accessed October 26, 2021).

two tragic incidents that occurred in two communities on the California coast, one was rated one of the 100 safest cities in America. Two young people who were having an acute mental health episode ended up dying at the hands of law enforcement when their parents and siblings called the police asking for help. Christine Goias called 9-1-1 seeking help for her son, Errol Chang, who was in the midst of a psychotic episode at his father's home. Police and the media arrived shortly after the call and spent 6 hours talking and working with Errol to get him out of the house. Errol's father disclosed there were weapons in the home and based on an established memorandum of understanding in the county, police were obligated to then call in the Special Weapons and Tactics (SWAT) team. The SWAT team engaged in repetitive communication and pointed weapons at the house and an individual experiencing paranoia. After 6 hours of communicating with the police, Errol was killed by specialized law enforcement agents 20 minutes after the SWAT team arrived. This happens to hundreds of families every year, Nihart stressed. Just 3 months later and 11 miles down the road, an 18-year-old woman with a developmental disability was refusing to take her medications. Her family called the police for help. The encounter with the county sheriff ended in the same result. There is an unsettling acceptance when individuals who have a mental illness and are experiencing a mental health crisis are killed, Nihart said.

In California, Jeannine Loucks, a psychiatric mental health clinical nurse specialist, collaborated with several organizations, she took all of the trainings that police received to prepare for these kinds of emergencies, modify the interventions, and created a series of videos that are now available to every police department in the country through the Orange County Mental Health Association. Nihart's community was able to acquire a psychological emergency response team that goes out with the police and gives families options on how to deal with their loved ones. "Imagine what could have happened in these two cases if 9-8-8 existed," said Nihart. "Imagine how we could help so differently, and imagine that this tragedy may not have had to occur at all."

THE 9-8-8 LIFELINE: POTENTIAL AND IMPLICATIONS FOR CRISIS RESPONSE

The Community Mental Health Services Framework

In communities today, dialing 9-1-1 typically provides one of three options: police, emergency medical services, or fire, but as Anita Everett, director of the Center for Mental Health Services at SAMHSA, explained, 9-1-1 systems for the most part are not setup to respond to mental health emergencies or to provide behavioral health services, even though a large proportion of 9-1-1 calls relate to mental health emergencies. In recognition of that fact Congress passed the National Suicide Hotline Designation Act of 2020, known colloquially as the 9-8-8 Act. As a result, in 2022, dialing 9-8-8 from any phone line (mobile phone, landline, or Voice over Internet Protocol line), will connect the caller with the National Suicide Prevention Lifeline.

Everett said that SAMHSA's Center for Mental Health Services, in its efforts to lower the national suicide rate, is working in four main areas. The first is to bring crisis response services into the twenty-first century so the entire mental health system is more responsive to the needs of individuals. Other components of SAMHSA's community mental health services framework include expanding the Zero Suicide program that was discussed on the first day of the workshop; enhancing suicide management skills among practicing health professionals; and providing more actionable data to local governments and health services organizations.

Regarding the first of those initiatives, Everett said that twenty-first century crisis services have three key components: a call, the mobile response for those who need it, and a place to go or someone to talk to, depending on the situation. Everett focused her discussion on the "someone to talk to" component.

Richard McKeon elaborated on how the 9-8-8 system will work. As Everett mentioned, the 9-8-8 system will build on the structure of the National Suicide Prevention Lifeline, which since 2005 has used the number 1-800-273-TALK (1-800-273-8255). Unlike 9-1-1 calls, 9-8-8 calls will all be directed to this national structure instead of being dispatched locally, said McKeon. Upon reaching 9-8-8, callers will hear a recorded message telling them to "press 1" if they are calling about a veteran or service member, which will then connect them to the veterans crisis line, or "press 2" if they need to be connected to a crisis counselor who is fluent in Spanish. Otherwise, the call will be distributed to one of the 184 local crisis centers located in every one of the 50 states as well as the territory of Guam. If the call is not answered within the first couple of minutes, it will go to a backup center; this is a feature that is not part of that the 9-1-1 system. McKeon added that the lifeline also has a small text chat service.

By July 2022 every phone system will need to make 9-8-8 operational, stated McKeon. Currently, most mobile phone systems have made 9-8-8 operational, but most landline systems have not, and the Federal Communications Commission (FCC) is proposing regulations to enable universal texting to 9-8-8. McKeon emphasized that this is a once-in-a-generation opportunity to improve mental health crisis services in America, both by expanding access to and awareness of connecting to 9-8-8, but also by being able to link to a more coordinated system that can connect people to the appropriate crisis intervention services. As part of this expansion, the Biden administration's budget released in May 2021 called for quadrupling funding for the National Suicide Prevention Lifeline to $102 million (SAMHSA, 2021).

McKeon added that SAMHSA is also working on the development of a comprehensive roadmap for 9-8-8 implementation, including providing more guidance for crisis centers and the states. The agency is also working to make sure that tribal communities are included and are able to receive the same crisis services. He concluded his remarks by noting that coordination between 9-8-8 and 9-1-1 will be important, as will educating the public about the differences between the two systems and when to call 9-8-8 versus 9-1-1.

Effectiveness of National Crisis Lines

National crisis lines were first highlighted in the 2012 Surgeon General's report *National Strategy for Suicide Prevention: Goals and Objectives for Action* (Office of the Surgeon General and National Action Alliance for Suicide Prevention, 2012), and they continued to have a prominent place in 2021 in the *Surgeon General's Call to Action to Implement the National Strategy for Suicide Prevention* (U.S. Surgeon General and National Action Alliance for Suicide Prevention, 2021), said Madelyn S. Gould, Irving Phillips Professor of Epidemiology in Psychiatry at the Columbia University Vagelos School of Physicians and Surgeons. However, she added, when the first national strategy was published in 2001, suicide crisis lines were not part of the strategy because the evidence for crisis line effectiveness was considered insufficient at the time.

What did happen in 2001, though, was SAMHSA's funding of a national network of local certified call centers that eventually became the National Suicide Prevention Lifeline. Equally important, SAMHSA has since funded continuous studies to evaluate the effectiveness of these crisis lines. "What has been unique to these evaluations and the relationship with SAMHSA and the lifeline is that these evaluation findings have been used to shape best practice standards across the network, with implementation of new standards then leading to additional evaluation studies" said Gould.

Prior to the lifeline evaluation, there was a pervasive impression that callers to crisis hotlines were not actually in a suicidal crisis, said Gould, but one of the major findings from 20 years of evaluation was to dispel this myth by demonstrating that individuals who are seriously contemplating suicide do call telephone crisis services (Gould et al., 2018; Kalafat et al., 2007). In addition, what Gould and her collaborators found in their first evaluation was that callers' suicide risk—the caller's intent to die, for example—was reduced significantly from the beginning to the end of the call (Gould et al., 2007). "So our original studies did show this reduction in suicide risk during the call," said Gould. Other evaluations have also found that counselors at lifeline centers are more likely to inquire about current suicidal ideation, recent ideation, and past attempts, and that callers are more likely to experience reduced distress at lifeline centers in comparison to some centers that were not part of the network. However, there is still room for improvement, less than half of National Suicide Prevention Lifeline centers inquire about recent suicide ideation or suicide attempts, suggesting a persistent problem among suicide (Ramchand et al., 2017).

She and her colleagues then started focusing on callers who were at imminent risk of suicide and found that crisis counselors were able to engage in collaboration with the callers to decide on an intervention in 76.4 percent of at-risk calls (Gould et al., 2016). "When you call the Lifeline, even if you are at an imminent-risk of suicide, the crisis counselors can collaborate," Gould explained. "They know how to collaborate with someone who is at imminent risk." For 19.1 percent of calls, the counselors did have to send emergency services, but they did so in collaboration with the caller (Gould et al., 2016). In 24.3 percent of imminent risk calls, she added, the counselors did have to send emergency services without the caller's collaboration (Gould et al., 2016), so overall, about 43 percent of imminent risk calls involve emergency services. In the collaborative interventions not involving emergency services, collaboration entailed involving a third party—a friend or family member—to eliminate access to lethal means (Gould et al., 2016).

Evaluation studies focused on types of interventions that can be carried out with third-party callers to protect the people who are at imminent risk. Such studies have shown that crisis counselors are able to provide a large range of interventions that can supplement, and at times replace, replace calling 9-1-1 (Gould et al., 2021b). Gould and her team have also done evaluation studies showing that follow-up calls from the crisis center do reduce suicidal individuals' perceived risk of future suicidal behavior (Gould et al., 2018).

To increase access to crisis services, lifeline services now have evolved to include not only telephone access but also crisis chat capability. Her team's evaluation of crisis chat functions found that almost 84 percent of people who chat report either current or recent suicidal ideation on a pre-chat survey, which is markedly higher than the estimated 23 percent of lifeline callers who are experiencing suicidal behavior on the day of or the day before their call (Gould et al., 2021a). Two-thirds of those individuals who used the chat function reported that the chat was helpful and that they were significantly and substantially less distressed at the end of the chat intervention than they were at the beginning, said Gould.

She said the time is now ripe for 9-8-8 because of the positive results of these evaluations. Gould also offered a number of suggested evaluations of the 9-8-8 system going forward. The questions to address include:

- To what extent is imminent risk reduced during the course of the crisis intervention without needing additional services?
- How often are 9-1-1 or police called by Lifeline crisis centers?

- How often are mobile crisis teams and stabilization units used?
- To what extent is information shared among Lifeline crisis centers, 9-1-1, emergency departments, and other crisis and emergency services?
- What outcomes emerge after different types of dispatch and information sharing?
- Do dispatch and outcomes vary for different ethnic, racial, and gender groups?

Veterans Crisis Line 9-8-8 Expansion Initiative and Implications

Lisa Kearney, director of the Veterans Crisis Line at the VA, spoke about the crisis line's current call volume and how the VA is preparing for the national rollout of the 9-8-8 system, particularly with regard to what happens after the call, text, or chat. The crisis line, she said, has fielded more than 5.4 million calls and 204,000 texts, engaged in more than 630,000 chats, and made more than 975,000 referrals since it opened in 2007. In fiscal year 2021, the crisis line has been answering around 2,000 calls per day, making more than 400 referrals per day on average, and dispatching emergency services just over 96 times per day on average. Compared to fiscal year 2020, average daily referrals and emergency dispatch calls are up by 14.6 percent and 20.0 percent, respectively.

VA has started two initiatives that align with preparing for 9-8-8. The Caring Letters initiative, said Kearney, is an evidence-based intervention for suicide prevention in which individuals who are in crisis have a follow-up letter sent at intervals to connect them with resources and provide them information about support they can receive (Reger et al., 2019). This program has been shown to help reduce the rate of suicide death, attempts, and ideation, and it has been added to the VA/U.S. Department of Defense clinical practice guidelines for addressing suicide risk. The Caring Letters initiative is now focused on expanding critical crisis intervention work to help veterans continue to feel supported and engaged, and the goal is to reach more than 90,000 veterans annually with nine letters over the course of a year after their call to the crisis line. Launched in June 2020, the crisis line has mailed more than 530,000 caring letters to more than 100,000 veterans. The VA is currently evaluating how effective this new program is at reducing suicide deaths, attempts, and ideation among veterans.

The second initiative, which the VA launched in June 2021, is the Peer Support Outreach whose mission is to provide support, hope, and recovery-oriented services to veterans who are identified as at increased risk for suicide. Kearney explained that this program provides care via phone and text messaging services to veterans who originally called the crisis line. VA peer specialists, who are veterans in recovery, staff the call center with supervision by licensed independent care providers. The goal is to support the veteran while he or she engages in follow-up care, either in the community or within the VA health system. "This is not just about getting people help within the moment of crisis, but getting them care, resources, and support afterwards to help them engage in follow-up," said Kearney.

Ongoing evaluation at the Peer Support Outreach Call Center has shown a 5-fold reduction in distress for callers at the end of the call than at the beginning, and callers are more likely to have less suicidal ideation at end of the call than the beginning. Callers were 91 percent less likely to have suicidal urgency at the end of the call compared to at the beginning, and 83 percent of callers reported feeling better following their call (Rasmussen et al., 2017). In addition, said Kearney, veterans were more likely to engage in care after receiving a responder referral (Britton et al., 2013).

Regarding the expected effects of the 9-8-8 rollout, Kearney said that the increased ease of accessing services should lead to increased call volumes and an increased need for collaboration and coordination after the call with services both internal and external to the VA. At a minimum, 9-8-8 has the potential to serve as a single point of entry into the care system for veterans, service members, and their families. She noted that the VA is preparing to expand its clinical operations and is currently increasing its quality assurance monitoring and beefing up its information technology infrastructure. In short, the VA expects 9-8-8 to increase access to the full continuum of care; this is driving the VA to consider how to shape and direct demand for mental health services to maximize capacity. As a final comment, she reminded everyone that while some carriers have already implemented 9-8-8, many have not, and individuals who subscribe to carriers that have not yet implemented it should still call 1-800-273-8255 and press 1 to reach the veterans crisis line, connect to chat at https://www.veteranscrisisline.net/get-help/chat, or connect via text at 838-255. These will remain active even after full activation of 9-8-8.

9-8-8 ROLLOUT: PRIVACY, CONFIDENTIALITY, AND EQUITY CONSIDERATIONS

The 9-8-8 Workforce and Culturally and Linguistically Appropriate Services

Sue Ann O'Brien, chief executive officer at Behavioral Health Link, said the advent of 9-8-8 will be transformational in helping people who are in a behavioral health crisis and getting them connected to care. Behavioral Health Link, she explained, operates Georgia's crisis and access line, which at the time of the workshop was on track to answer more than 250,000 calls in 2021, as well as texts and chats.

O'Brien noted that the key to success with the 9-8-8 rollout will be providing callers with access to the full continuum of care so they receive the care that is right for them. "The predictions are that the call volume will drastically increase with the ease of the three-digit number, and that is a great thing in terms of accessibility and [it is hoped] decreased stigma, but we will have to have those other services in place," she said. She added that if the full range of options is not available, the result will be a continued overreliance on 9-1-1, with individuals ending up in jail, the emergency department, or the morgue. "These adverse outcomes are exponentially more likely for people of color," said O'Brien.

Ensuring a sufficient workforce to meet the expected increase in demand will be an essential component for providing access to the full spectrum of care, and building that workforce cannot rely solely on licensed clinicians because they are already in short supply. Moreover, the majority of the behavioral health workforce in the United States is approximately 85 percent White according to some estimates, while the number of non-White residents is approaching half of the U.S. population, with about 57 million people speaking a language other than English in their homes. These demographics got O'Brien thinking about the National Standards for Culturally and Linguistically Appropriate Services (CLAS) that HHS released in 2000 and updated in 2013. The National Standards for CLAS, she reminded the audience, are a set of 15 recommendations for health care agencies that was intended to advance health equity and to eliminate health care disparities in health care organizations.

One of the recommendations is to have a workforce that proportionately represents the population being served (HHS, 2013), which O'Brien said is an issue that many organizations, including hers, have been looking at, especially with the recent and ongoing civil unrest and attention to racial injustice. In Atlanta, where Blacks account for 51 percent of the population, her call center workforce is 77 percent Black. However, the population outside of Atlanta is more than 60 percent White, which can make it difficult for callers to connect with trained call center staff because of cultural and life experience differences as well, she said. "I think what is needed is more of an emphasis on cultural humility," said O'Brien, who defined cultural humility as the ability to maintain an interpersonal stance that is open to the aspects of cultural identity most important to the person. "If we cannot bridge that divide, it might indeed be a matter of life and death," she said. "It is imperative that we leverage a well-trained, diverse, and even nonclinical workforce, including peer support specialists, if we are truly going to address the equity issue head-on."

PATIENT-CENTERED CARE CONSIDERATIONS IN CRISIS SERVICES FOR AMERICAN INDIAN/ALASKA NATIVE PEOPLE

The IHS provides health care to 2.2 million American Indians and Alaska Natives living in 37 states, including Alaska, with an intentional focus on the culture of each of the more than 500 unique tribal communities with which IHS works, said End of Horn. IHS approaches equity within health care—providing needed health care, when it is needed, and how it is needed—from a perspective of humanization in health care. What this entails, said End of Horn, is the use of a person-centered approach that asserts the intrinsic dignity of all human beings through the adoption of core values that include honesty and integrity, caring compassion, altruism, empathy, and respect for others (Velasco Bueno and La Calle, 2020).

Patient-centered care, explained End of Horn, focuses on accepting, assessing, and identifying patients from their perspective, as well as understanding what the patient needs and empowering them to go where they want to go to address their needs (Cheraghi et al., 2017). Factors that play a role in implementing patient-centered care include open visitation policies; communication; a focus on the well-being of the patient; having the presence and participation of relatives; care for the health care professional; prevention, management and monitoring; having humanized architecture and infrastructure, and providing appropriate end-of-life care (Velasco Bueno and La Calle, 2020).

In many tribal communities, the act of sharing stories is seen as medicine, said End of Horn. Patient-centered care in that context requires the health care provider to listen to the individual as they share what is happening to them and what they are experiencing; this can involve a translator for those individuals who feel more comfortable telling their story in their native language. "Including family, communication, relationship building, being open to cultural influences, and providing traditional treatment options allows Western medicine to meet the needs of Native people," she said (Sylliboy and Hovey, 2020).

Providing culturally humble, aware, and appropriate care comes down to building capacity, said End of Horn. Building capacity, she explained, is a fundamental component to the community-level development of outcomes that use the community's resources to address problems and issues. Building capacity requires including strong representation of the Native community in creating community-based interventions and education and developing networks throughout the community (Smith-Morris and Epstein, 2014). Intensive outreach, as well as implementing services in equal partnership with the community, are essential for success, she emphasized.

BUILDING EQUITY INTO THE FRONT END OF 9-8-8

Victor Armstrong, director of the Division of Mental Health, Developmental Disabilities, and Substance Abuse Services in the North Carolina Department of Health and Human Services, said the 9-8-8 rollout is a tremendous opportunity to create a system where equity is the foundation rather than an afterthought. He noted equity is not just about race, culture, and ethnicity. Armstrong said,

> The lens of equity is about the intersectionality of race, culture, and ethnicity, in addition to living with mental health challenges. It is about being Black and living with a serious mental illness. It is about being Latino and living with intellectual disability resulting from traumatic brain injury. It is about being Native American and living with a substance use disorder. It is about being an Asian trans-person struggling with an anxiety disorder exacerbated by the discrimination that often accompanies mental illness, the hatred that is perpetrated toward trans Americans, and the increasing rates of violence toward Asian Americans.

Armstrong contends that the very construct of the current U.S. mental health care system is flawed, beginning with its response to individuals experiencing mental health emergencies. The current system, he said, was not built from the perspective of individuals with lived health experiences, nor was it designed to address their mental health needs. "I would argue that our current system is not designed to protect and nurture the individual experiencing the mental health emergency, but to protect the rest of us from the individual experiencing the mental health emergency, and that is wrong," said Armstrong. "The introduction of 9-8-8 will provide us an opportunity to mitigate those challenges and to correct that wrong." Because many people of color do not have access to outpatient services or crisis services in the communities where they live, their introduction to the mental health care system often ends up being in the back of a police car or in an acute care emergency department when they are in a state of crisis, and "that is not conducive to good clinical outcomes, nor is it likely to foster a positive relationship with the mental health system," said Armstrong. Research indicates that Black adults more likely to report psychological stressors than their White counterparts (SAMHSA, 2020; Williams, 2018), but they are less likely to enter treatment and more likely to terminate treatment prematurely (Williams, 2018), said Armstrong.

He explained that suicide itself is not a disease, but rather the worst possible outcome of a combination of many complex factors. That being the case, there are opportunities to intervene with person-centered approaches before a person reaches the point of suicidality. Suicide prevention, however, should be about more than detaining someone when they are in crisis. Assessing risk at the individual level or the community level, said Armstrong, involves considering not only risk factors but also protective factors.

In addition, without understanding or acknowledging the effect of cultural beliefs, including stigma; the relationships with law enforcement; or the effect of structural racism on an individual's life and their perception of their place in America, an intervention may become another traumatic experience that the individual will have to carry. On the other hand, he added, building cultural humility in the system via 9-8-8 will increase the likelihood that individuals receive care in their communities and that they receive care that accounts for the intersectionality of race, ethnicity, culture, and sexual identity.

Systemic racism and bias, both explicit and implicit, are multilayered and seep into every crevice of society, including law enforcement, schools, and health care, and the mental health system is not immune, said Armstrong, adding,

> But we know that inequity exists, and it is our moral responsibility to address those inequities by leaning into equity in every decision that we make as clinicians, policy makers, or simply as change agents. Either lean into creating a more equitable system or perpetuate inequity.

Armstrong pointed out that according to the Washington Post Police Shooting Database, 6,697 people have been shot and killed by a police officer in the line of duty since January 1, 2015. Nearly one-fourth were Black and almost 97 percent of those were Black males (*The Washington Post*, 2021). People in mental health crisis are at high risk of death during a police interaction, with 23 percent of people killed by police identified as having a mental illness. He cited those figures not to impugn officers but to suggest that there is a flaw in the system, one that puts Black individuals who are having a mental health crisis, whether a psychotic episode or suicidality, at high risk of a negative outcome.

However, 9-8-8 can be the spark that dismantles racism in a mental health response system and become a building block in creating a system that is more equitable, said Armstrong. It can do so by supporting the creation of more mental health resources in communities of color and underserved communities. Those resources, he noted, can include mobile crisis care, facility-based crisis care, peer respite, and others designed to divert individuals away from emergency departments and jails. Armstrong said,

> We can create more community-based resources that provide access to upstream treatment rather than continuing in the crisis response mode that we have existed in for the past several decades, and we can seize the opportunity to build a workforce that mirrors the populations served.

While Blacks comprise roughly 13 percent of America's population, only about 4 percent of American psychologists are Black, and only about 2 percent of America's psychiatrists are Black, Armstrong noted.

There is a ready-made but under used workforce of individuals from a broad range of racial, ethnic, and cultural groups with lived mental health experience, said Armstrong. In North Carolina, there are approximately 4,000 trained peer specialists, though only some 1,600 are gainfully employed. "We need to utilize the peer workforce, pay them a living wage, and build them into our crisis continuum to respond to individuals experiencing mental health emergencies at a time when they most need someone who understands their immediate challenges," adding

> We can increase the percent of historically marginalized populations receiving behavioral health services by building and earning trust between historically marginalized communities, behavioral health care providers, and funders as we bring them to the table in planning our 9-8-8 model.

It is possible, he stated, to reimagine the nation's approach to mental health and build an equitable mental health care system. The challenge is to seize the opportunity afforded by the 9-8-8 rollout to work with community partners and community media to:

- create grassroots messaging to educate communities, combat stigma, and address concerns about receiving mental health treatment;
- use expertise and care providers of color who have traditionally served historically marginalized communities, often without access to government grants and contracts; and
- engage them in the planning, giving voice to those with lived experience.

Indeed, without paying attention to the intersectionality of clinical expertise and the voice of historically marginalized individuals, any approach will be ill advised, ill informed, and ill fated, said Armstrong. Listening only to the opinions of intellectuals, the desires of legislators, and the needs of the majority would create a system that might work for 80 percent of the U.S. population but not address the needs of 80 percent of the Black, Latinx, or Native American population, he added. "If you have not lived the life experience of those you seek to assist and do not have decision makers with that life experience at the table, you cannot fully understand the challenges and address the need, no matter how well intentioned you may be," said Armstrong.

Historically marginalized communities, whether marginalized because of race, ethnicity, or diagnosis, are not looking to be rescued, nor are they looking for a handout, he noted. Rather, historically marginalized communities are looking for a collaborative partner who will value their expertise and life experience. "Those living with mental health challenges, those struggling with addictions, and those living with intellectual disabilities or traumatic brain injuries are themselves a historically marginalized population, and they are looking for an opportunity to have their voices be heard" said Armstrong.

In closing, Armstrong reiterated that implementing the 9-8-8 system creates an opportunity to build a more equitable and responsive system, one that is not only evidence based and evidence informed but informed by the community and individuals' lived experiences. "My life experience tells me that if we do not build equity into 9-8-8 on the front end, the most powerless and vulnerable among us will not receive equity, justice, or access to the mental health resources they need and deserve," he said.

BUILDING CULTURAL COMPETENCE WITHIN CRISIS SERVICES

A Potential Framework for Developing Culturally Responsive and Personalized Evidence-Based Mental Health Interventions for Culturally Diverse Populations

May Yeh, associate professor of psychology at San Diego State University, described the PersIn Approach to developing personalized, evidence-based interventions for culturally diverse populations (McCabe et al., 2020). This approach entails three steps. The first step is the identification of factors and dimensions upon which personalization for culturally diverse populations might need to occur. This is a critical step, said Yeh, because individual health care providers may not be aware of the different cultural dimensions that might affect care for any given person. In their work, she and colleagues accomplished this step by finding factors or dimensions that have published research showing a relationship to clinically meaningful outcomes, have variability across cultural groups, and can be addressed through personalization.

In the case of suicide prevention, clinically meaningful outcomes might relate to service use, engagement with the intervention, or a reduction in suicide-related ideation or behavior. The types of cultural factors that may be relevant, said Yeh, may vary based upon the clinically relevant outcome. For example, when considering barriers to using mental health services, stigma may be a stronger barrier in certain cultural groups, while mistrust of care providers or lack of access—or knowledge of—services may be a more important barrier for another.

She also noted that when assessing risk and protective factors for suicidal behavior, Joyce Chu and colleagues indicate that it may be important to account for cultural factors such as family conflict, social discord, acculturative stress, minority stress, cultural sanctions related to suicide, and idioms of distress (Chu et al., 2020). Ascertaining clinically and culturally relevant dimensions may require further research, literature review, and consultation with experts, community members, and leaders or other stakeholders, added Yeh.

The second step of the PersIn framework focuses on finding ways to briefly assess the components identified in the first step, recognizing that that groups are heterogeneous. It may be, for example, that certain factors are more salient for some individuals within a group or may apply to others outside of that group. In addition, people may affiliate with more than one cultural group. "Developing assessments for the specific dimensions or factors allows us to broaden the ability of the intervention to respond to different groups while also individualizing the treatment protocol to the specific person," said Yeh. Results of this brief assessment, she explained, gives care providers a sense of the factors that may be especially important to address with a particular individual before they begin the intervention.

In the third step, tools or modifications are developed to address the dimensions or factors identified in the first step. For example, one tool might be developed to address a potential risk factor of family conflict, while another tool may be constructed to address minority-related stress. As she explained, developing these tools for the array of possibilities gives care providers a toolbox containing what they may need to address important factors. There is also a need to train care providers in effective use of these tools.

Once the personalized intervention is developed, it is used as follows: the brief assessment can be given before the intervention begins, and the tools or modifications are triggered and then implemented to personalize intervention. The goal, said Yeh, is to provide a culturally responsive intervention that takes into account important cultural dimensions while making it possible to standardize the use of the tools and personalize the intervention to an individual when implemented.

BEYOND CULTURAL COMPETENCY

Culture is a value-laden term, with values themselves being a reflection of culture, said End of Horn. She noted that anthropologically, there is no set definition of culture, but there are three aspects to the concept: a group of people who "belong together" by value of some shared features, a systemic organizer of psychological systems of individual persons, and how the person and environment are interrelated (Valsiner, 2003). In other words, culture is not just systemic beliefs, practices, or knowledge, but rather culture is what belongs to a group of people and to what those people belong. This conceptualization of culture says not to lump all American Indians and Alaska Natives into one group because that takes away from the individuality and uniqueness of each tribal nation, said End of Horn.

Cultural competency is not a clinical skill, said End of Horn. Rather, it is an opportunity for individuals to learn about local customs and local perspectives, to build networks, and to incorporate those elements and aspects into the care that is provided and allow the care to be responsive to the community needs and political patterns, especially when talking about tribal nations. Tribal nations change often with regard to administration and political pattern, she said, and so providing services that are understanding of that and responsive to that will go to where the patient is, deliver what they need, and provide equitable health care (Smith-Morris and Epstein, 2014). "I cannot stress this enough: you have to go to the community and become part of that community in order to provide services," said End of Horn, adding

> This is not something that the community should be coming to you for. You should be going to the community, inviting them in, building bridges, and working to understand their reality and then incorporating that within the services that you're providing, because no one person is going to be able to provide that.

In closing, emphasized that she is just one person from just one of the 500 federally recognized tribes and 100 more state-recognized tribes, each of which has different realities. "So please consider going beyond cultural competency and see it as an opportunity," said End of Horn.

WORKING IN DIVERSE COMMUNITIES

Jennifer Battle, director of access with the Harris Center for Mental Health and Intellectual/Developmental Disabilities, began her comments by saying that she wishes she could have specific training for every single community represented, not just in Harris County but the entire state of Texas, but the likelihood of that happening is slim. As a result, the focus on cultural humility is key if the 9-8-8 call centers are going to be able to work collaboratively with the numerous communities throughout the state and be able to connect callers with support in their specific community.

Harris County, home to Houston, has almost 5 million people, with 69 percent of the residents identifying as coming from a community of color. More than 145 languages are spoken, and almost half of the county's residents either speak a language other than English or are bilingual. "That's exciting as a community but terrifying from a call center perspective," said Battle.

One topic of discussion regarding health equity has been around how to handle calls from a non-native English speaker and where the responsibility of the 9-8-8 system morphs into the community's responsibility to provide language assistance. The discussions have also raised the possibility of training the people who provide translation services to serve in the call centers because they may not have expertise or understanding around mental health issues or suicide prevention.

Battle encouraged audience members who are not involved in their 9-8-8 planning grant process to reach out to their local crisis centers so they can find out what is going on and see if there is anything they can do to lend their expertise and voice to that process, especially if their work has a strong equity focus. She then noted that conversations at the state level have focused on suicide prevention as a form of social justice work, saying

> The more that we can create a life worth living for people, the more that people are going to reach out for the care that they need when they need it, and hopefully trust us enough to be able to be the folks that they reach out to.

As a final comment, she reiterated the call to involve local communities in whatever plans are being made, as well as to reach out to local call centers and support them however possible.

LATINX YOUTH AND THE UNDOCUMENTED

Thomas Chávez, associate professor in counseling psychology at the University of New Mexico, noted that the Latinx population is the second largest racial or ethnic group in the United States, representing about 60.6 million people, 80 percent of whom are U.S. citizens. The Latinx community includes many diverse groups, with most immigrants coming from Colombia, Guatemala, and Honduras, followed by El Salvador, Cuba, and the Dominican Republic. The smallest immigrant Latinx group comes from Mexico, he added.

One theory about Latinx well-being centers on acculturation, where the longer an immigrant stays and aligns with U.S. values and health systems, the poorer their health outcomes are. Chávez said the measure of acculturation should take into consideration affective, cognitive, and behavioral dimensions to understand its effect on health. It is also important, he said, to consider the sociological systems that affect well-being, such as whether the individual came to the United States as a child or whether they migrated as an adolescent or young adult. Another contextual feature is the diversity of the destination culture; migrating to an area with less diversity makes it more likely that the individual will experience stress. In particular, Chávez explained, there are two types of acculturative stress, including the pressure to assimilate as well as stress resulting from discrimination. Youth also experience the complex developmental stressors typical for adolescence, as well as bullying that often coincides with anti-immigrant sentiments that may be present in a particular region. Such stresses may contribute to internalizing and externalizing behaviors.

Chávez said there are lower rates of death by suicide in the Latinx population compared to other ethnic and racial groups (Ramchand et al., 2021), though Latino youth are more likely to report suicidal ideation and attempts than their non-Hispanic peers (Limas and Vaughn, 2018; Silva and Van Orden, 2018). Latina groups report elevated rates of experiencing violence and oppression related to their gender, particularly in regard to cultural expressions that are in discord with their acculturation (Zayas and Pilat, 2008), said Chávez. In fact, Latina adolescents are more likely to attempt suicide when they have poor psychosocial functioning and family crisis. Suicide rates among LGBTQIA+ Latinx youth are also elevated even after accounting for depression and substance use (Boyas et al., 2019).

Understanding the Latinx population has been limited to theoretical perspectives and has not considered their unique experiences, said Chávez. Critical race theory, a methodology for helping investigators maintain consciousness of racialized constructs and historical sociopolitical mechanisms, can help investigators and practitioners understand such experiences (Ford and Airhihenbuwa, 2010).

LatCrit, or Latino critical theory, allows investigators to examine how multiple forms of oppression can intersect with the lives of people of color and how interactions manifest in day-to-day experiences unique to the Latinx community, such as immigration status, language, ethnicity, and culture (Bernal, 2002). Another useful theory, UndocuCrit or Undocumented critical theory, offers a critical approach for analyzing how racist immigrant practices, policies, and rhetoric function to spread fear among populations of undocumented immigrants (Aguilar, 2018).

For example, his team has used critical race theory to inform a study in which they found that Latinx young adults and their families avoided health care institutions for fear of being reported to immigration officials and were constantly stressed because of financial and emotional issues connected to the lack of health insurance and having to pay for care out of pocket. This population, he noted, largely depends on community health clinics for all their health care needs and only seek emergency services when faced with a life or death situation. This study also identified risk factors for suicidal behaviors that included exposure to violence and trauma, acculturation of absent family systems, social and linguistic isolation, economic stress, and family conflict. Protective factors included the values of familism, personalism, and respect; parental interventions, highlighting and promoting biculturalism and bilingualism, and expanding social networks (Chávez et al., 2021).

Chávez suggested focusing suicide prevention efforts on social media campaigns to reduce stigma of mental health and substance use disorders and to promote safety, as well as enforcing nondiscrimination laws, guaranteeing universal coverage for all youth, implementing trauma-informed policies, keeping families together, and promoting community resiliency. He emphasized the need to promote mental health from a young age and to include antibullying training. In addition, he noted the importance of evidence-based practices for Latinx behavioral health and the creation of partnerships among family, community, and schools to promote resilience and heal trauma.

BUILDING CULTURAL COMPETENCE WITHIN CRISIS SERVICES

Xinzhi Zhang, chief of health inequities and the global health branch of the National Heart, Lung, and Blood Institute, noted that suicide is the leading cause of death among Asian American adolescents (Murphy et al., 2021). A number of factors are contributing to this rise, said Zhang, including family conflict, intergenerational differences, lack of English proficiency, self-image and identity issues, bullying, discrimination because of Asian names, and academic pressures.

To counter these factors, the U.S. Public Health Service, SAMHSA, the National Institute on Minority Health and Health Disparities, and the Asian American Health Initiative in Montgomery County, Maryland, started a Healthy Mind Initiative that is reaching out to different Asian communities to increase awareness and promote suicide prevention among Asian adolescents. This initiative relies on individuals from the various communities who speak the language and understand the specific culture. He noted that getting that type of community engagement involvement will be critical for implementing 9-8-8 initiatives.

Zhang concluded his comments with an example of the type of program that has come out of this initiative. In 2019, students 16 to 18 years old competed in a national essay contest to speak up about mental health (NIMH, 2021). The "This is My Story" competition received more than 200 essays from 34 states and Puerto Rico, with 10 receiving awards and 2 receiving honorable mentions. A second competition is in the works, said Zhang.

9-8-8, HEALTH EQUITY, AND FAITH WITHIN THE BLACK COMMUNITY

Brandon Johnson, public health advisor to SAMHSA's Center for Mental Health Services, discussed how 9-8-8 can be used to improve outcomes for Black youth, who have twice the suicide rate of White youth and among whom those rates have been increasing at an alarming rate, as Lindsey discussed during the first webinar. The rollout of the 9-8-8 system, said Johnson, could address health equity issues by increasing access to mobile crisis teams for Black families, which in turn could save lives by avoiding engagement with law enforcement. He noted, too, that local crisis centers often have information on local mental health resources and community supports. Connecting Black and Brown families with culturally appropriate resources increases the likelihood for engagement and would benefit youth specifically if equipped with resources designed to meet their needs.

It is important as well to remember the family. "As we talk about young Black children between the ages of 5 and 12, we are talking about a family unit," said Johnson, adding,

> Often, it will be the parents reaching out to 9-8-8 asking for resources, wanting to know what they can do for their youth, and as we know, there has been structural racism and systemic racism that has made it more difficult for Black families to thrive.

It is also critical to have resources dedicated to the specific social determinants of health that make it more difficult for a family to access various services. There is also the need to have resources for LGBTQIA+ youth, youth who are experiencing homelessness, those in foster care, and others.

Johnson said that 9-8-8 creates the opportunity to address the specific needs of various populations, to use the available data, and create resources that are timely and relevant. Moreover, by emphasizing cultural humility, it should be possible to understand those aspects of the lived experience that may be driving suicidal behavior but may not have been accounted for and attended to in the past.

As co-leader of the Faith Communities Task Force, which leads the National Action Alliance for Suicide Prevention's efforts to engage faith communities in suicide prevention, Johnson said that a focus on faith communities can:

- help integrate and coordinate suicide prevention activities across multiple sectors and settings,
- increase knowledge about the factors that offer protection from suicidal behaviors and that promote wellness and recovery, and
- provide care and support to individuals affected by suicide deaths and attempts to promote healing and implement community strategies to help prevent further suicides.

Involving faith communities in suicide prevention efforts can also help people get connected to services and coordinate their care, as well as help educate individuals about mental health and how it can affect them. "As we engage with faith communities, we understand that the communities oftentimes are already doing this type of work in promoting hope and healing, as well as making linkages to services and instilling in individuals an increased sense of purpose," said Johnson.

As 9-8-8 rolls out, he said it will be important to reach out to faith leaders, engage with them, and help them understand the potential benefits it can bring to their communities so they can in turn convey that information to their communities. Engaging faith communities in these conversations can normalize the conversation about mental health and remove some of the stigma around accessing mental health services.

Toward that end, Johnson and his colleagues will be working with faith communities to help them if they want to develop specific dissemination materials for the rollout of 9-8-8. He noted that the faith communities he has engaged with are eager to be helpful and want to know how to best support individuals to lead their best lives possible. The task force is also creating dialogs and holding informational sessions and webinars with faith leaders across the country to answer questions and be available for individuals to ask what they can do to help.

A HISTORIC FIRST: SPECIALIZED SERVICES IN 9-8-8 FOR LGBTQIA+ YOUTH

LGBTQIA+ youth are at high risk of suicidal ideation, said Sam Brinton (they/them), vice president of advocacy and government affairs at the Trevor Project. Data collected by the National Survey on LGBTQIA+ Youth Mental Health show that 42 percent of LGBTQIA+ youth overall seriously considered suicide in the past year, but Brinton noted that there were differences in suicide risk among different populations of LGBTQIA+ youth. While 12 percent of White LGBTQIA+ youth attempted suicide, 31 percent of Native and Indigenous LGBTQIA+ youth, 21 percent of Black and multiracial LGBTQIA+ youth, and 18 percent of Latinx LGBTQIA+ youth attempted suicide in the past year.

Brinton also noted that 94 percent of LGBTQIA+ youth said that recent policies had negatively affected their mental health. But Brinton said 9-8-8 is a tremendous advance because the legislation requires an implementation plan for what are called "specialized services" for high-risk populations, including LGBTQIA+ youth, as well as minority and rural populations. Brinton also noted that when the legislation passed both houses of Congress by unanimous vote, it was the first and only time an LGBTQIA+-inclusive bill passed without a single no vote.

ENSURING 9-8-8 SERVES ALL

Tracie Schneider, Deaf Services Coordinator for the Arkansas Department of Health and Human Services, said the 9-8-8 initiative will neither be truly inclusive nor fully accessible unless text message and direct video call acceptance capabilities are integrated into the rollout. Currently, she said, people with disabilities have to deal with multiple phone numbers—a text number, a teletypewriter (TTY) number, a speech-to-speech number, and others—to reach crisis services, so one important goal of the 9-8-8 rollout is to make sure that everyone has only one number to remember and that it responds to text or video calls without any extra steps.

As it is now envisioned, a Deaf person who primarily uses American Sign Language (ASL) would have to access the 9-8-8 crisis line through what is called a video relay service, which uses either standalone equipment or smartphone/desktop apps to place a call using an interpreter over a broadband connection. "If I am trying to call 9-8-8, I have to facilitate that through an interpreter because texting to 9-8-8 is not available," said Schneider. The same is true, she said, for direct video calling that would automatically direct the call to someone who knows ASL. Not only would direct video call acceptance be linguistically affirming, but it would also be culturally appropriate as well, she noted.

INCLUDING SCHOOLS IN THE CRISIS RESPONSE SYSTEM

Sharon Hoover, professor and co-director of the National Center for School Mental Health at the University of Maryland School of Medicine, said it is imperative for the nation to build a universal system for behavioral health promotion and early identification and intervention to minimize crises while simultaneously addressing the failings of the current crisis response system for children. Such a system for children should include schools because one of the most central tenets to creative, accessible, and equitable systems of crisis care and behavioral health care is to meet people where they are.

Hoover noted that an increasing number of schools are installing what many are referring to as *comprehensive school mental health systems*, which are partnerships between the education and behavioral health sectors to support a full continuum of mental health supports and services, including mental health promotion and treatment. These comprehensive school mental health systems, she explained, provide a full array of supports that can include promoting positive mental health for all students, providing prevention interventions for those students who are most at risk for developing mental health conditions or mental health challenges, and providing early intervention services for those students who may screen positive for mental health concerns. She added that when treatment is provided in school settings, young people are far more likely to not only be identified early but to initiate and complete care.

The new National Center for Safe Supportive Schools,[21] funded by SAMHSA, focuses on three areas: developing comprehensive school mental

---

[21] Additional information is available at https://www.ncs3.org (accessed November 5, 2021).

health systems, implementing culturally responsive and equitable policies, and supporting trauma-informed, healing-centered practices.

Hoover said,

> It is increasingly evident to educators and to the mental health field that for all students to feel safe and supported in schools and to support their behavioral health and well-being, we must not only put mental health supports and services in place, but also ensure that all of our approaches are culturally responsive, antiracist, and equitable, and that they are delivered through a trauma-informed and healing-centered approach.

An essential component of comprehensive school mental health systems is crisis prevention and response. In fact, said Hoover, implementing comprehensive, multitiered systems of mental health support in schools has been demonstrated to reduce emotional and behavioral health crises (Bohnenkamp et al., 2021; Kase et al., 2017; SAMHSA and CMS, 2019; Stephan et al., 2015). Her team, for example, recently finished a 5-year implementation and study of crisis prevention and response that included peer training for students from various social groups in each school who were trained in conflict management and bullying prevention, as well as online virtual simulation technology to train teachers on how to support students experiencing psychological distress, as well as clear referral, assessment, and coordination processes and a structured process for post-crisis prevention. Positive outcomes from this program included 56 percent fewer suspensions in the intervention schools, 76 percent fewer office referrals, and more on-site crisis response as opposed to off-site referrals to emergency departments or law enforcement (Bohnenkamp et al., 2021). As a final comment, she urged everyone to keep children, adolescents, and young adults in mind as the nation rolls out its 9-8-8 system.

DISCUSSION: HEALTH EQUITY AND 9-8-8

Pearson posed a question from the audience asking if calls to 9-8-8 are actually free and if it is accessible to people in Canada. McKeon replied that all calls to 9-8-8 are toll free, with the cost absorbed by SAMHSA's lifeline grant program. Geographically, 9-8-8 will be accessible across all 50 states and all U.S. territories, but not in Canada. The Public Health Agency of Canada and the Mental Health Commission of Canada have been in contact with SAMHSA with regard to developing a similar system for Canada. Pearson noted that the U.S. 9-8-8 system is modeled after the United Kingdom's system, and McKeon added that some—North Dakota, Connecticut, Maryland, Colorado, and Georgia—have their own three-digit crisis lines in operation. Presumably, those will continue to operate, but discussions about what will happen to those systems going forward are important, says McKeon.

Pearson commented that while it is important to have these crisis services in place, the best outcome would be to have fewer crises. She then asked the panelists for their suggestions regarding upstream interventions. McKeon responded that there needs to be an increased awareness that intervening with someone in crisis is different from what needs to be done to prevent someone from becoming suicidal in the first place. In his view, there are three levels of intervention strategies: those that can help prevent people from becoming suicidal, those that can prevent individuals who are having suicidal thoughts from progressing to an acute suicidal crisis, and those such as 9-8-8 that can help someone at imminent risk.

Brinton said that the message needs to be promoted by encouraging people to call 9-8-8 during a very bad day, saying,

> If we are doing our job as a nation, then ... we can answer that phone or that text message quickly and efficiently and let you know that we are spending time with you, that you are not alone. That is the major preventive activity in this work.

Brinton noted that not every state legislature has passed legislation on 9-8-8 implementation yet, but they emphasized that every school should have a suicide prevention policy and that every teacher, faith community leader, and mental health professional should know about 9-8-8 and spread the word about it so that calling it becomes a normalized process.

REFLECTIONS: OPPORTUNITIES TO BUILD INCLUSIVE CARE STRUCTURES

To conclude the workshop, Barbara Limandri, a psychiatric nurse with the American Psychiatric Nurses Association and professor emerita at Linfield University, and David Covington, chief executive officer and president of RI International and a partner with Behavioral Health Link, offered their thoughts and reflections. Limandri first commented that 9-8-8 is a long overdue community intervention for suicide prevention that will make it easier to ask for help. However, she added that 9-8-8 is not a cure-all. "We still have to reduce stigma," she said.

Limandri noted that suicide is the equivalent of a heart attack in terms of an emergency, and that while it took a few decades, cardiopulmonary resuscitation (CPR) is now a community intervention. In her mind, suicide prevention is mental health CPR, and everyone needs to be trained in the basics. The good news, she said, is that robust research on suicide intervention and prevention shows that the skills for suicide prevention are simple: asking the question, "Are you thinking of killing yourself?"; listening to the response without judgment; and then connecting that person to those who can help them. This skill, called QPR, or question, persuade, and refer, should be taught to everyone along with CPR, Limandri said.

What the public needs to recognize, she said, is that suicide prevention is effective. "Suicidal thinking and behaviors are a transient state of extreme impulsivity and lack of perspective," said Limandri. "Having someone else step in and be a source of hope and perspective can be an immense improvement in the struggle for the person with suicidal thinking and behaviors." What this comes down to, she said, is seeing each person in their setting and culture and taking care of them. She also pointed out that family, friends, and neighbors are the most essential first responders in a suicide crisis, not the mental health professional. Limandri said, "We get them after they are in the crisis, after they have made an attempt, but it is the neighbor, the family member that is hearing it first, and they do not know what to do." However, they can learn those skills in the same way that community members learn CPR she added. As a final comment, she called for a systemic approach to suicide prevention. "I think the COVID pandemic has taught us that our health care system and our mental health care system are broken, and we need to improve on that as well," said Limandri. She also posted two resources for suicide prevention training:

- Psychiatric-Mental Health Nurse Essential Competencies for Assessment and Management of Individuals at Risk for Suicide (https://www.apna.org/i4a/pages/index.cfm?pageid=5684)
- Question, Persuade, and Refer (https://qprinstitute.com)

Covington noted that the ideal crisis system for mental health, addiction, and suicidal behavior may seem like a fanciful dream, but the United States created the 9-1-1 system to respond to emergencies, just as it is about to do for the 9-8-8 system and mental health emergencies. Currently, however, a common experience for a person on their worst day is that they perceive what happens as punishment, not care or support. They are detained, delayed, and denied care, and they spend time in hospital emergency departments—and some people who are having a mental health crisis end up handcuffed in the back of a police vehicle.

Nonetheless, the combination of the pressure from the COVID-19 pandemic on hospitals, discussions of race inequity, a reconsideration of the role of law enforcement in this process, and the galvanizing promise of 9-8-8 provides an opportunity to create something different for everyone in crisis, but particularly for people of color and the LGBTQIA+ community. "This is an amazing day and once-in-a-lifetime opportunity to transform mental health care," said Covington.

REFERENCES

Aarons, G. A., M. Hurlburt, and S. M. Horwitz. 2011. Advancing a conceptual model of evidence-based practice implementation in public service sectors. *Administration and Policy in Mental Health and Mental Health Services Research* 38(1):4-23.

Aarons, G. A., A. E. Green, L. A. Palinkas, S. Self-Brown, D. J. Whitaker, J. R. Lutzker, J. F. Silovsky, D. B. Hecht, and M. J. Chaffin. 2012. Dynamic adaptation process to implement an evidence-based child maltreatment intervention. *Implementation Science* 7(1):32.

Aguilar, C. 2018. Undocumented critical theory. *Cultural Studies ↔ Critical Methodologies* 19(3):152-160.

Ali, B., I. R. H. Rockett, T. R. Miller, and J. B. Leonardo. 2021. Racial/ethnic differences in preceding circumstances of suicide and potential suicide misclassification among US adolescents. *Journal of Racial and Ethnic Health Disparities.* https://doi.org/10.1007/s40615-020-00957-7.

Anestis, M. D., A. E. Bond, S. E. Daruwala, S. L. Bandel, and C. J. Bryan. 2021. Suicidal ideation among individuals who have purchased firearms during COVID-19. *American Journal of Preventive Medicine* 60(3):311-317.

Avery, A., M. Landen, T. Massaro, C. Novak, D. Sanchez, and A. Sandoval. 2018. *2020–2022 new mexico state health improvement plan.* Santa Fe, NM: New Mexico Department of Health.

Bahraini, N., L. A. Brenner, C. Barry, T. Hostetter, J. Keusch, E. P. Post, C. Kessler, C. Smith, and B. B. Matarazzo. 2020. Assessment of rates of suicide risk screening and prevalence of positive screening results among us veterans after implementation of the Veterans Affairs suicide risk identification strategy. *JAMA Network Open* 3(10):e2022531.

Bernal, D. D. 2002. Critical race theory, latino critical theory, and critical raced-gendered epistemologies: Recognizing students of color as holders and creators of knowledge. *Qualitative Inquiry* 8(1):105-126.

Bohnenkamp, J. H., C. M. Schaeffer, R. Siegal, T. Beason, M. Smith-Millman, and S. Hoover. 2021. Impact of a school-based, multi-tiered emotional and behavioral health crisis intervention on school safety and discipline. *Prevention Science* 22(4):492-503.

Boyas, J. F., T. Villarreal-Otálora, L. R. Alvarez-Hernandez, and M. Fatehi. 2019. Suicide ideation, planning, and attempts: The case of the Latinx LBG youth. *Health Promotion Perspectives* 9(3):198-206.

Bray, M. J. C., N. O. Daneshvari, I. Radhakrishnan, J. Cubbage, M. Eagle, P. Southall, and P. S. Nestadt. 2021. Racial differences in statewide suicide mortality trends in Maryland during the coronavirus disease 2019 (COVID-19) pandemic. *JAMA Psychiatry* 78(4):444-447.

Bridge, J. A., S. C. Marcus, and M. Olfson. 2012. Outpatient care of young people after emergency treatment of deliberate self-harm. *Journal of the American Academy of Child and Adolescent Psychiatry* 51(2):213-222.

Bridge, J. A., L. Asti, L. M. Horowitz, J. B. Greenhouse, C. A. Fontanella, A. H. Sheftall, K. J. Kelleher, and J. V. Campo. 2015. Suicide trends among elementary school-aged children in the United States from 1993 to 2012. *JAMA Pediatrics* 169(7):673-677.

Bridge, J. A., L. M. Horowitz, C. A. Fontanella, A. H. Sheftall, J. Greenhouse, K. J. Kelleher, and J. V. Campo. 2018. Age-related racial disparity in suicide rates among US youths from 2001 through 2015. *JAMA Pediatrics* 172(7):697-699.

Britton, P., R. Bossarte, C. Thompson, J. Kemp, and K. Conner. 2013. Influences on call outcomes among veteran callers to the national veterans crisis line. *Suicide & Life-Threatening Behavior* 43.

Burstein, B., H. Agostino, and B. Greenfield. 2019. Suicidal attempts and ideation among children and adolescents in US emergency departments, 2007–2015. *JAMA Pediatrics* 173(6):598-600.

Cantrell, C., S. Valley-Gray, and R. E. Cash. 2012. Suicide in rural areas: Risk factors and prevention. In *Rural mental health: Issues, policies, and best practices*, edited by K. B. Smalley, J. C. Warren, and J. P. Rainer. New York: Springer. Pp. 213-228.

CDC (Centers for Disease Control and Prevention). 2019. *Youth risk behavior survey: Data summary & trends report 2009–2019*. https://www.cdc.gov/healthyyouth/data/yrbs/pdf/YRBSDataSummaryTrendsReport2019-508.pdf (accessed November 4, 2021).

CDC. 2021a. *National Center for Injury Prevention and Control. Web-based Injury Statistics Query and Reporting System (WISQARS)*. https://www.cdc.gov/injury/wisqars (accessed November 16, 2021).

CDC. 2021b. *National Violent Death Reporting System (NVDRS), violence prevention*. https://www.cdc.gov/violenceprevention/datasources/nvdrs/index.html (accessed November 4, 2021).

Chávez, T., S. Vences, Y. Ruiz, J. Navarro, F. Rodriguez, and I. Aranda. 2021. Critical incidences in U.S. health care systems experienced by undocumented young adults. *Health Equity* 5:569-576.

Cheraghi, M. A., M. Esmaeili, and M. Salsali. 2017. Seeking humanizing care in patient-centered care process: A grounded theory study. *Holistic Nursing Practice* 31(6):359-368.

Children's Hospital Colorado. 2021. *Children's Hospital Colorado declares a state of emergency for youth mental health*. https://www.childrenscolorado.org/about/news/2021/may-2021/youth-mental-health-state-of-emergency (accessed November 4, 2021).

Chu, J., B. Maruyama, H. Batchelder, P. Goldblum, B. Bongar, and R. E. Wickham. 2020. Cultural pathways for suicidal ideation and behaviors. *Cultural Diversity & Ethnic Minority Psychology* 26(3):367-377. https://doi.org/10.1037/cdp0000307 (accessed November 16, 2021).

Coleman, B. W., and Congressional Black Caucus Emergency Taskforce on Black Youth Suicide and Mental Health. 2019. *Ring the alarm: The crisis of Black youth suicide in America*. Washington, DC: Congressional Black Caucus Emergency Taskforce on Black Youth Suicide and Mental Health.

Costello, E. J., J. P. He, N. A. Sampson, R. C. Kessler, and K. R. Merikangas. 2014. Services for adolescents with psychiatric disorders: 12-month data from the National Comorbidity Survey-Adolescent. *Psychiatric Services* 65(3):359-366.

Craig, S. L., L. B. McInroy, A. D. Eaton, G. Iacono, V. W. Y. Leung, A. Austin, and C. Dobinson. 2019. An affirmative coping skills intervention to improve the mental and sexual health of sexual and gender minority youth (Project Youth Affirm): Protocol for an implementation study. *JMIR Research Protocols* 8(6):e13462.

Cummings, J. R., N. A. Ponce, and V. M. Mays. 2010. Comparing racial/ethnic differences in mental health service use among high-need subpopulations across clinical and school-based settings. *Journal of Adolescent Health* 46(6):603-606.

Czeisler, M., R. I. Lane, E. Petrosky, J. F. Wiley, A. Christensen, R. Njai, M. D. Weaver, R. Robbins, E. R. Facer-Childs, L. K. Barger, C. A. Czeisler, M. E. Howard, and S. M. W. Rajaratnam. 2020. Mental health, substance use, and suicidal ideation during the COVID-19 pandemic—United States, June 24–30, 2020. *Morbidity and Mortality Weekly Report* 69(32):1049-1057.

Damschroder, L. J., D. C. Aron, R. E. Keith, S. R. Kirsh, J. A. Alexander, and J. C. Lowery. 2009. Fostering implementation of health services research findings into practice: A consolidated framework for advancing implementation science. *Implementation Science* 4(1):50.

Dobscha, S. K., K. D. Clark, S. Newell, E. A. Kenyon, E. Karras, J. A. Simonetti, and M. Gerrity. 2021. Strategies for discussing firearms storage safety in primary care: Veteran perspectives. *Journal of General Internal Medicine* 36(6):1492-1502.

Eylem, O., L. de Wit, A. van Straten, L. Steubl, Z. Melissourgaki, G. T. Danışman, R. de Vries, A. J. F. M. Kerkhof, K. Bhui, and P. Cuijpers. 2020. Stigma for common mental disorders in racial minorities and majorities a systematic review and meta-analysis. *BMC Public Health* 20(1):879.

Fontanella, C. A., D. L. Hiance-Steelesmith, G. S. Phillips, J. A. Bridge, N. Lester, H. A. Sweeney, and J. V. Campo. 2015. Widening rural-urban disparities in youth suicides, United States, 1996–2010. *JAMA Pediatrics* 169(5):466-473.

Ford, C. L., and C. O. Airhihenbuwa. 2010. Critical race theory, race equity, and public health: Toward antiracism praxis. *American Journal of Public Health* 100(Suppl 1):S30-S35.

GAO (U.S. Government Accountability Office). 2018. *Discipline disparities for Black studnets, boys, and students with disabilities*. Washington, DC: GAO. https://www.gao.gov/assets/gao-18-258.pdf (accessed November 4, 2021).

GAO. 2019. *Opportunities exist for VA to better identify and address racial and ethnic disparities*. Washington, DC: GAO.

Gennetian, L. A., S. Wolf, H. D. Hill, and P. A. Morris. 2015. Intrayear household income dynamics and adolescent school behavior. *Demography* 52(2):455-483. https://doi.org/10.1007/s13524-015-0370-9.

Gennetian, L., R. Seshadri, N. Hess, A. Winn, and R. Goerge. 2016. Supplemental Nutrition Assistance Program (SNAP) benefit cycles and student disciplinary infractions. *Social Service Review* 90:403-433.

Goldman-Mellor, S., M. Olfson, C. Lidon-Moyano, and M. Schoenbaum. 2019. Association of suicide and other mortality with emergency department presentation. *JAMA Network Open* 2(12):e1917571.

Gould, M., J. Kalafat, J. Harrismunfakh, and M. Kleinman. 2007. An evaluation of crisis hotline outcomes part 2: Suicidal callers. *Suicide and Life-Threatening Behavior* 37:338-352.

Gould, M. S., A. M. Lake, J. L. Munfakh, H. Galfalvy, M. Kleinman, C. Williams, A. Glass, and R. McKeon. 2016. Helping callers to the National Suicide Prevention Lifeline who are at imminent risk of suicide: Evaluation of caller risk profiles and interventions implemented. *Suicide and Life-Threatening Behavior* 46(2):172-190.

Gould, M. S., A. M. Lake, H. Galfalvy, M. Kleinman, J. L. Munfakh, J. Wright, and R. McKeon. 2018. Follow-up with callers to the National Suicide Prevention Lifeline: Evaluation of callers' perceptions of care. *Suicide and Life-Threatening Behavior* 48(1):75-86.

Gould, M. S., S. Chowdhury, A. M. Lake, H. Galfalvy, M. Kleinman, M. Kuchuk, and R. McKeon. 2021a. National Suicide Prevention Lifeline crisis chat interventions: Evaluation of chatters' perceptions of effectiveness. *Suicide and Life-Threatening Behavior.* http://doi.org/10.1111/sltb.12795 (accessed November 16, 2021).

Gould, M. S., A. M. Lake, M. Kleinman, H. Galfalvy, and R. McKeon. 2021b. Third-party callers to the National Suicide Prevention Lifeline: Seeking assistance on behalf of people at imminent risk of suicide. *Suicide and Life-Threatening Behavior.* http://doi.org/10.1111/sltb.12769 (accessed November 16, 2021).

Green, A. E., C. E. Willging, M. M. Ramos, D. Shattuck, and L. Gunderson. 2018. Factors impacting implementation of evidence-based strategies to create safe and supportive schools for sexual and gender minority students. *Journal of Adolescent Health* 63(5):643-648.

Harris, J., E. Wahesh, M. Barrow, and J. Fripp. 2021. Demographics, stigma, and religious coping and Christian African Americans' help seeking. *Counseling and Values* 66:73-91.

Hays, K., and K. D. Lincoln. 2017. Mental health help-seeking profiles among African Americans: Exploring the influence of religion. *Race and Social Problems* 9(2):127-138.

Hedegaard, H., S. C. Curtin, and M. Warner. 2021. *Suicide mortality in the United States, 1999–2019.* Hyattsville, MD: National Center for Health Statistics.

HHS (U.S. Department of Health and Human Services). 2013. *National standards for culturally and linguistically appropriate services in health and health care: A blueprint for advancing and sustaining CLAS policy and practice.* https://thinkculturalhealth.hhs.gov/assets/pdfs/EnhancedCLASStandardsBlueprint.pdf (accessed November 16, 2021).

Hogg, B., J. C. Medina, I. Gardoki-Souto, I. Serbanescu, A. Moreno-Alcázar, A. Cerga-Pashoja, E. Coppens, M. D. Tóth, N. Fanaj, B. A. Greiner, C. Holland, K. Kõlves, M. Maxwell, G. Qirjako, L. de Winter, U. Hegerl, V. Pérez-Sola, E. Arensman, and B. L. Amann. 2021. Workplace interventions to reduce depression and anxiety in small and medium-sized enterprises: A systematic review. *Journal of Affective Disorders* 290:378-386.

Hom, M. A., and I. H. Stanley. 2021. Considerations in the assessment of help-seeking and mental health service use in suicide prevention research. *Suicide and Life-Threatening Behavior* 51(1):47-54.

Horowitz, L. M., D. Snyder, E. Ludi, D. L. Rosenstein, J. Kohn-Godbout, L. Lee, T. Cartledge, A. Farrar, and M. Pao. 2013. Ask suicide-screening questions to everyone in medical settings: The asQ'em Quality Improvement Project. *Psychosomatics* 54(3):239-247.

Ivey-Stephenson, A. Z., Z. Demisssie, A. E. Crosby, D. M. Stone, E. Gaylor, N. Wilkins, R. Lowry, and M. Brown. 2020. Suicidal ideation and behaviors among high school students—Youth Risk Behavior Survey, United States, 2019. *Morbidity and Mortality Weekly Report* 69(1):47-59.

Jaycox, L. H., J. A. Cohen, A. P. Mannarino, D. W. Walker, A. K. Langley, K. L. Gegenheimer, M. Scott, and M. Schonlau. 2010. Children's mental health care following Hurricane Katrina: A field trial of trauma-focused psychotherapies. *Journal of Trauma and Stress* 23(2):223-231.

Kalafat, J., M. Gould, J. Munfakh, and M. Kleinman. 2007. An evaluation of crisis hotline outcomes part 1: Nonsuicidal crisis callers. *Suicide and Life-Threatening Behavior* 37:322-337.

Kase, C., S. Hoover, G. Boyd, K. D. West, J. Dubenitz, P. A. Trivedi, H. J. Peterson, and B. D. Stein. 2017. Educational outcomes associated with school behavioral health interventions: A review of the literature. *Journal of School Health* 87(7):554-562.

Klonsky, E. D., and A. May. 2015. The three-step theory (3st): A new theory of suicide rooted in the "ideation-to-action" framework. *International Journal of Cognitive Therapy* 8:114-129.

Layman, D. M., J. Kammer, E. Leckman-Westin, M. Hogan, J. Goldstein Grumet, C. D. Labouliere, B. Stanley, J. Carruthers, and M. Finnerty. 2021. The relationship between suicidal behaviors and zero suicide organizational best practices in outpatient mental health clinics. *Psychiatric Services* https://ps.psychiatryonline.org/doi/10.1176/appi.ps.202000525 (accessed November 16, 2021).

LeCloux, M. A., M. Weimer, S. L. Culp, K. Bjorkgren, S. Service, and J. V. Campo. 2020. The feasibility and impact of a suicide risk screening program in rural adult primary care: A pilot test of the ask suicide-screening questions toolkit. *Psychosomatics* 61(6):698-706.

LESC (Legislative Education Study Committee). 2021a. *School-based health care*. Legislative Education Study Committee Bill Analysis, 55th Legislature, 1st Session, 2021. https://www.nmlegis.gov/Sessions/21%20Regular/LESCAnalysis/SM015.PDF (accessed November 5, 2021).

LESC. 2021b. *Full-time school nurse. Legislative Education Study Committee Bill Analysis*. 55th Legislature, 1st Session, 2021. https://www.nmlegis.gov/Sessions/21%20Regular/LESCAnalysis/SB0031.PDF (accessed November 5, 2021).

LFC (Legislative Finance Committee). 2021. *Full-time nurse in every school, HB 32. Fiscal Impact Report*. https://nmlegis.gov/Sessions/19%20Regular/bills/house/HB0476.pdf (accessed November 5, 2021).

Limas, E. A., and E. L. Vaughan. 2018. Associations between substance use disorders and suicidal ideation: An investigation of latino emerging adults. *Emerging Adulthood* 7(1):21-30.

Lindsey, M. A., C. L. Barksdale, S. F. Lambert, and N. S. Ialongo. 2010. Social network influences on service use among urban, African American youth with mental health problems. *Journal of Adolescent Health* 47(4):367-373.

Lindsey, M. A., A. H. Sheftall, Y. Xiao, and S. Joe. 2019. Trends of suicidal behaviors among high school students in the United States: 1991–2017. *Pediatrics* 144(5):e20191187.

Lyons, V. H., M. J. Haviland, D. Azrael, A. Adhia, M. A. Bellenger, A. Ellyson, A. Rowhani-Rahbar, and F. P. Rivara. 2021. Firearm purchasing and storage during the COVID-19 pandemic. *Injury Prevention* 27(1):87-92.

McCabe, K. M., M. Yeh, and A. A. Zerr. 2020. Personalizing behavioral parent training interventions to improve treatment engagement and outcomes for culturally diverse families. *Psychological Research and Behavior Management* 13:41-53.

McGuire, T. G., and J. Miranda. 2008. New evidence regarding racial and ethnic disparities in mental health: Policy implications. *Health Affairs (Project Hope)* 27(2):393-403.

Merikangas, K. R., J. P. He, M. Burstein, J. Swendsen, S. Avenevoli, B. Case, K. Georgiades, L. Heaton, S. Swanson, and M. Olfson. 2011. Service utilization for lifetime mental disorders in U.S. adolescents: Results of the National Comorbidity Survey-Adolescent Supplement (NCS-A). *Journal of the American Academy of Child and Adolescent Psychiatry* 50(1):32-45.

Michelmore, L., and P. Hindley. 2012. Help-seeking for suicidal thoughts and self-harm in young people: A systematic review. *Suicide and Life-Threatening Behavior* 42(5):507-524.

Mishara, B. L., and S. Stijelja. 2020. Trends in US suicide deaths, 1999 to 2017, in the context of suicide prevention legislation. *JAMA Pediatrics* 174(5):499-500.

Misra, S., V. W. Jackson, J. Chong, K. Choe, C. Tay, J. Wong, and L. H. Yang. 2021. Systematic review of cultural aspects of stigma and mental illness among racial and ethnic minority groups in the United States: Implications for interventions. *American Journal of Community Psychology* https://doi.org/10.1002/ajcp.12516 (accessed November 16, 2021).

Murphy, S. L., J. Xu, K. D. Kochanek, E. Arias, and B. Tejada-Vera. 2021. Deaths: Final data for 2018. *National Vital Statistics Reports* 69(13). https://www.cdc.gov/nchs/data/nvsr/nvsr69/nvsr69-13-508.pdf (accessed November 29, 2021).

National Action Alliance for Suicide Prevention: Transforming Communities-Community-Based Suicide Prevention Priority Group. 2017. *Transforming communities: Key elements for the implementation of comprehensive community-based suicide prevention.* Washington, DC: National Action Alliance for Suicide Prevention.

Nazroo, J. Y., K. S. Bhui, and J. Rhodes. 2020. Where next for understanding race/ethnic inequalities in severe mental illness? Structural, interpersonal and institutional racism. *Sociology of Health & Illness* 42(2):262-276.

Nelson, H. D., L. M. Denneson, A. R. Low, B. W. Bauer, M. O'Neil, D. Kansagara, and A. R. Teo. 2017. Suicide risk assessment and prevention: A systematic review focusing on veterans. *Psychiatric Services* 68(10):1003-1015.

Newell, S., E. Kenyon, K. D. Clark, V. Elliott, A. Rynerson, M. S. Gerrity, E. Karras, J. A. Simonetti, and S. K. Dobscha. 2021. Veterans are agreeable to discussions about firearms safety in primary care. *Journal of the American Board of Family Medicine* 34(2):338.

NIMH (National Institute of Mental Health). 2021. NIH Announces Winners of High School Mental Health Essay Contest. https://www.nimh.nih.gov/news/science-news/2019/nih-announces-winners-of-high-school-mental-health-essay-contest (accessed November 16, 2021).

Office of the Surgeon General and National Action Alliance for Suicide Prevention. 2012. *2012 national strategy for suicide prevention: Goals and objectives for action.* Washington, DC: HHS.

Oransky, M., E. Z. Burke, and J. Steever. 2019. An interdisciplinary model for meeting the mental health needs of transgender adolescents and young adults: The Mount Sinai Adolescent Health Center approach. *Cognitive and Behavioral Practice* 26(4):603-616.

Pistone, I., U. Beckman, E. Eriksson, H. Lagerlöf, and M. Sager. 2019. The effects of educational interventions on suicide: A systematic review and meta-analysis. *International Journal of Social Psychiatry* 65(5):399-412.

Ramchand, R., L. Jaycox, P. Ebener, M. L. Gilbert, D. Barnes-Proby, and P. Goutam. 2017. Characteristics and proximal outcomes of calls made to suicide crisis hotlines in California. *Crisis* 38(1):26-35.

Ramchand, R., J. A. Gordon, and J. L. Pearson. 2021. Trends in suicide rates by race and ethnicity in the united states. *JAMA Network Open* 4(5):e2111563.

Ramos, M. M., C. Greenberg, R. Sapien, J. Bauer-Creegan, B. Hine, and C. Geary. 2013. Behavioral health emergencies managed by school nurses working with adolescents. *Journal of School Health* 83(10):712-717.

Rasmussen, K. A., D. A. King, M. S. Gould, W. Cross, W. Tang, K. Kaukeinen, X. Tu, and K. L. Knox. 2017. Concerns of older veteran callers to the veterans crisis line. *Suicide and Life-Threatening Behavior* 47(4):387-397.

Ream, G. L. 2020. An investigation of the LGBTQ+ youth suicide disparity using national violent death reporting system narrative data. *Journal of Adolescent Health* 66(4):470-477.

Reger, M. A., H. M. Gebhardt, J. M. Lee, B. A. Ammerman, R. P. Tucker, B. B. Matarazzo, A. E. Wood, and D. A. Ruskin. 2019. Veteran preferences for the caring contacts suicide prevention intervention. *Suicide and Life-Threatening Behavior* 49(5):1439-1451.

Rhodes, A. E., M. Sinyor, M. H. Boyle, J. A. Bridge, L. Y. Katz, J. Bethell, A. S. Newton, A. Cheung, K. Bennett, P. S. Links, L. Tonmyr, and R. Skinner. 2018. Emergency department presentations and youth suicide: A case-control study. *Canadian Journal of Psychiatry* 64(2):88-97.

Richards, J. E., S. D. Hohl, C. D. Segal, D. C. Grossman, A. K. Lee, U. Whiteside, C. Luce, E. J. Ludman, G. Simon, R. B. Penfold, and E. C. Williams. 2021. "What will happen if I say yes?" perspectives on a standardized firearm access question among adults with depressive symptoms. *Psychiatric Services* 72(8):898-904.

Ritchie, M. J., K. M. Dollar, C. J. Miller, J. L. Smith, K. A. Oliver, B. Kim, S. L. Connolly, E. Woodward, T. Ochoa-Olmos, S. Day, J. A. Lindsay, and J. E. Kirchner. 2020. *Using implementation facilitation to improve healthcare (version 3)*. Washington, DC: Veterans Health Administration.

Riva, J. J., K. M. Malik, S. J. Burnie, A. R. Endicott, and J. W. Busse. 2012. What is your research question? An introduction to the PICOT format for clinicians. *Journal of the Canadian Chiropractic Association* 56(3):167-171.

Robinson, W. L., C. R. Whipple, L. A. Jason, and C. E. Flack. 2021. African American adolescent suicidal ideation and behavior: The role of racism and prevention. *Journal of Community Psychology* 49(5):1282-1295.

Ruch, D. A., A. H. Sheftall, P. Schlagbaum, J. Rausch, J. V. Campo, and J. A. Bridge. 2019. Trends in suicide among youth aged 10 to 19 years in the United States, 1975 to 2016. *JAMA Network Open* 2(5):e193886.

Russon, J., R. Washington, A. Machado, L. Smithee, and J. Dellinger. 2021. Suicide among LGBTQIA+ youth: A review of the treatment literature. *Aggression and Violent Behavior* 101578.

SAMHSA (Substance Abuse and Mental Health Services Administration). 2020. *Serious psychological distress in the past year among adults 18 years of age and over, percentage, 2019. Results from the 2019 National Survey on Drug Use and Health: Mental Health Detailed Tables*. Table 10.43B. Rockville, MD: SAMHSA.

SAMHSA. 2021. *SAMHSA awards Vibrant Emotional Health the grant to administer 988 dialing code for the National Suicide Prevention Lifeline.* SAMHSA News Release. https://www.samhsa.gov/newsroom/press-announcements/202106161430 (accessed November 4, 2021).

SAMHSA and CMS (Centers for Medicare & Medicaid Services). 2019. Guidance to states and school systems on addressing mental health and substance use issues in schools. In *Joint Informational Bulletin*. Washington, DC: SAMHSA and CMS.

Searles, V. B., M. A. Valley, H. Hedegaard, and M. E. Betz. 2014. Suicides in urban and rural counties in the United States, 2006–2008. *Crisis* 35(1):18-26.

Shattuck, D., J. L. Hall, A. Green, C. Greenberg, L. Peñaloza, M. Ramos, and C. Willging. 2020. Recruitment of schools for intervention research to reduce health disparities for sexual and gender minority students. *Journal of School Nursing* 36(4):258-264.

Shattuck, D., R. Sebastian, M. Ramos, and K. Zamarin. 2021. *Behavioral health emergencies managed by school nurses*. Paper presented at National Association of School Nurses 2021 Virtual, Transforming Student Health: School Nurses Leading the Way.

Silva, C., and K. A. Van Orden. 2018. Suicide among hispanics in the United States. *Current Opinion in Psychology* 22:44-49.

Simonetti, J. A., B. Dorsey Holliman, R. Holliday, L. A. Brenner, and L. L. Monteith. 2020. Correction: Firearm-related experiences and perceptions among United States male veterans: A qualitative interview study. *PLOS ONE* 15(4):e0231493.

Simonetti, J., D. Azrael, W. Zhang, and M. Miller. 2021. *Normative beliefs among veteran firearm owners regarding when clinicians should discuss firearm safety with patients: Results from the 2019 National Firearms Survey*. Paper presented at U.S. Department of Veterans Affairs/U.S. Department of Defense National Suicide Prevention Conference.

Smith-Morris, C., and J. Epstein. 2014. Beyond cultural competency: Skill, reflexivity, and structure in successful tribal health care. *American Indian Culture and Research Journal* 38:29-48.

Stapelberg, N. J. C., J. Sveticic, I. Hughes, A. Almeida-Crasto, T. Gaee-Atefi, N. Gill, D. Grice, R. Krishnaiah, L. Lindsay, C. Patist, H. V. Engelen, S. Walker, M. Welch, S. Woerwag-Mehta, and K. Turner. 2021. Efficacy of the zero suicide framework in reducing recurrent suicide attempts: Cross-sectional and time-to-recurrent-event analyses. *British Journal of Psychiatry* 219(2):427-436.

Stephan, S. H., G. Sugai, N. Lever, and E. Connors. 2015. Strategies for integrating mental health into schools via a multitiered system of support. *Child and Adolescent Psychiatric Clinics of North America* 24(2):211-231.

Sylliboy, J. R., and R. B. Hovey. 2020. Humanizing Indigenous peoples' engagement in health care. *Canadian Medical Association Journal* 192(3):E70.

Terrell, S. 2019. *Film explores 2013 behavioral health shakeup in New Mexico*. AP News. https://apnews.com/article/08a5ed186c424b01a1cae3b95fd679bb (accessed November 5, 2021).

U.S. Surgeon General and National Action Alliance for Suicide Prevention. 2021. *The Surgeon General's call to action to implement the National Strategy for Suicide Prevention*. Washington, DC: HHS. https://www.hhs.gov/sites/default/files/sprc-call-to-action.pdf (accessed November 4, 2021).

VA (U.S. Department of Veterans Affairs). 2019. *National veteran suicide prevention annual report*. Washington, DC: VA.

Valsiner, J. 2003. Culture and its transfer: Ways of creating general knowledge through the study of cultural particulars. *Online Readings in Psychology and Culture* 2(1).

Velasco Bueno, J. M., and G. H. La Calle. 2020. Humanizing intensive care: From theory to practice. *Critical Care Nursing Clinics of North America* 32(2):135-147.

Walrath, C., L. G. Garraza, H. Reid, D. B. Goldston, and R. McKeon. 2015. Impact of the Garrett Lee Smith Youth Suicide Prevention Program on suicide mortality. *American Journal of Public Health* 105(5):986-993.

The Washington Post. 2021. *Washington Post police shooting database.* https://www.washingtonpost.com/graphics/investigations/police-shootings-database (accessed November 4, 2021).

While, D., H. Bickley, A. Roscoe, K. Windfuhr, S. Rahman, J. Shaw, L. Appleby, and N. Kapur. 2012. Implementation of mental health service recommendations in England and Wales and suicide rates, 1997–2006: A cross-sectional and before-and-after observational study. *Lancet* 379(9820):1005-1012.

Whiteside, C. 2019. *Health behaviors and conditions of adult New Mexicans, results from the New Mexico Behavioral Risk Factor Surveillance System (BRFSS) 2019 annual report.* Santa Fe, NM: New Mexico Department of Health.

Whiteside, C., and D. Green. 2021. *Sexual orientation and gender identity: Data from the youth risk and resiliency survey and behavioral risk factor surveillance system.* Santa Fe, NM: New Mexico Department of Health.

WHO (World Health Organization). 2014. *Preventing suicide: A global imperative.* Geneva, Switzerland: WHO Press.

Willging, C. E., and E. M. Trott. 2018. Outsourcing responsibility: State stewardship of behavioral health care services. In *Unequal coverage: The experience of health care reform in the United States*, edited by J. Mulligan and H. Castaneda. New York: New York University Press. Pp. 231-253.

Willging, C. E., A. E. Green, and M. M. Ramos. 2016. Implementing school nursing strategies to reduce LGBTQ adolescent suicide: A randomized cluster trial study protocol. *Implementation Science* 11(1):145.

Willging, C., M. Kano, A. E. Green, R. Sturm, M. Sklar, S. Davies, and K. Eckstrand. 2020. Enhancing primary care services for diverse sexual and gender minority populations: A developmental study protocol. *BMJ Open* 10(2):e032787.

Williams, D. R. 2018. Stress and the mental health of populations of color: Advancing our understanding of race-related stressors. *Journal of Health and Social Behavior* 59(4):466-485.

Zayas, L. H., and Pilat, A. M. 2008. Suicidal behavior in Latinas: explanatory cultural factors and implications for intervention. *Suicide & Life-Threatening Behavior* 38(3):334-342.

Appendix A

Statement of Task

A planning committee of the National Academies of Sciences, Engineering, and Medicine will organize and host a virtual public workshop through two webinars that will explore strategies and interventions to counter the rising prevalence of suicide. The workshop will feature invited presentations and moderated discussions on topics that may include:

- The scope of the public health problem, with a focus on patterns of suicidal ideation, suicide attempts, and death by suicide
- The current data on the increasing prevalence of death by suicide, such as
  - methods of death by suicide (firearm, suffocation, poisoning, other);
  - variations in death by suicide rates across ethnic and racial groups as well as among veterans, military personnel, and other high-risk groups such as workers in certain occupations;
  - key factors related to increased risk of suicide; and
  - the impact of COVID-19 pandemic on rates of suicide
- What is known about the effectiveness of approaches and interventions to reduce harm and prevent risk of suicide
  - factors that increase resilience among vulnerable populations
  - understanding stigma and its impact on access to care
- Policy opportunities to support, improve, and implement early interventions and expand access to care among vulnerable populations with specific needs
- Areas where further research is needed to address gaps in evidence

The planning committee will develop the agenda for the workshop sessions, select and invite speakers and discussants, and moderate the discussions. A proceedings of the presentations and discussions at the workshop will be prepared by a designated rapporteur in accordance with institutional guidelines.

Appendix B

Workshop Agenda

Strategies and Interventions to Reduce Suicide: A Two-Part Virtual Workshop

AGENDA

U.S. SUICIDE SUBGROUP TRENDS: OPPORTUNITIES IN HEALTH CARE TO REDUCE SUICIDE RISK
TUESDAY, JUNE 22, 2021
1:00–3:30 PM ET

WELCOME FROM THE FORUM ON MENTAL HEALTH AND SUBSTANCE USE DISORDERS

1:00 PM   **Mary Roary, Ph.D.**
Director, Office of Behavioral Health Equity
Office of Intergovernmental and External Affairs
Office of the Assistant Secretary for Mental Health and Substance Use
Substance Abuse and Mental Health Services Administration

Matt Tierney, M.S., APRN
President, American Psychiatric Nurses Association
Clinical Professor, University of California, San Francisco, School of Nursing

Clinical Director of Substance Use Treatment and Education,
University of California, San Francisco, Office of Population
Health
Planning Committee Co-Chairs

CHOOSING HOPE OVER SUICIDE

1:10 PM **Kevin Hines**
Suicide Survivor, Storyteller, Filmmaker

SESSION 1
SUICIDE TRENDS IN U.S. SUBGROUPS

1:20 PM *Session 1 Moderator:*
Jane Pearson, Ph.D.
Special Advisor to the Director on Suicide Research
National Institute of Mental Health
National Institutes of Health
Planning Committee Member

Speakers:
Jeff Bridge, Ph.D.
Director, Center for Suicide Prevention and Research
Abigail Wexner Research Institute
Nationwide Children's Hospital

Crystal L. Barksdale, Ph.D., M.P.H.
Acting Deputy Director
Chief, Minority Mental Health Research
Office for Disparities Research and Workforce Diversity
National Institute of Mental Health
National Institutes of Health

SESSION 1
PANEL DISCUSSION AND AUDIENCE Q&A

1:40 PM *Panelists:*
Holly C. Wilcox, Ph.D.
Professor, Johns Hopkins Bloomberg School of Public Health
Johns Hopkins University School of Medicine
Johns Hopkins University School of Education

Richard McKeon, Ph.D.
Chief, Suicide Prevention Branch
Division of Prevention, Traumatic Stress, and Special Programs
Center for Mental Health Services
Substance Abuse and Mental Health Services Administration

Crystal L. Barksdale, Ph.D., M.P.H.
Acting Deputy Director
Chief, Minority Mental Health Research
Office for Disparities Research and Workforce Diversity
National Institute of Mental Health
National Institutes of Health

Jeff Bridge, Ph.D.
Director, Center for Suicide Prevention and Research
Abigail Wexner Research Institute
Nationwide Children's Hospital

SESSION 2A
EXPERIENCES IN IMPLEMENTING SUICIDE PREVENTION CARE IN FEDERAL HEALTH CARE SETTINGS

2:00 PM   *Session 2 Moderator:*
Andrew Moon, Psy.D.
Associate Director, Education and Training
Suicide Prevention Program
Office of Mental Health and Suicide Prevention
U.S. Department of Veterans Affairs
Planning Committee Member

Speakers:
Lisa Brenner, Ph.D.
Professor, University of Colorado
Director, Rocky Mountain Mental Illness Research, Education, and Clinical Center
Vice Chair, Department of Physical Medicine and Rehabilitation
U.S. Department of Veterans Affairs

Joseph Simonetti, M.D., M.P.H.
Physician and Suicide Prevention Researcher
Rocky Mountain Mental Illness Research Education
    and Clinical Center for VA Suicide Prevention
University of Colorado

Pamela End of Horn, M.S.W., LICSW
National Suicide Prevention Consultant,
Division of Behavioral Health
Office of Clinical and Preventive Services
Indian Health Service

SESSION 2B
IMPROVING SUICIDE PREVENTION: ADDRESSING KNOWN BARRIERS TO HEALTH CARE ACCESS

2:30 PM *Session 2 Moderator:*
Ursula Whiteside, Ph.D.
Chief Executive Officer, NowMattersNow.org
Clinical Faculty, University of Washington

Speakers:
Cathleen Willging, Ph.D.
Center Director and Senior Research Scientist
Pacific Institute for Research and Evaluation
Southwest Center

Lisa Brenner, Ph.D.
Professor, University of Colorado
Director, Rocky Mountain Mental Illness Research,
    Education, and Clinical Center
Vice Chair, Department of Physical Medicine and
    Rehabilitation
U.S. Department of Veterans Affairs

Michael Lindsey, Ph.D., M.S.W., M.P.H.
Executive Director, Silver's McSilver Institute for
    Poverty Policy and Research
New York University

SESSION 2
PANEL DISCUSSION AND AUDIENCE Q&A

3:15 PM *Moderator:*
Erin Bagalman, M.S.W.
Director, Division of Behavioral Health Policy
Office of Behavioral Health, Disability, and Aging Policy
Office of the Assistant Secretary for Planning and Evaluation
U.S. Department of Health and Human Services
Planning Committee Member

Panelists:
Lisa Brenner, Ph.D.
Professor, University of Colorado
Director, Rocky Mountain Mental Illness Research, Education, and Clinical Center
Vice Chair, Department of Physical Medicine and Rehabilitation
U.S. Department of Veterans Affairs

Pamela End of Horn, M.S.W., LICSW
National Suicide Prevention Consultant,
Division of Behavioral Health
Office of Clinical and Preventive Services
Indian Health Service

Michael Lindsey, Ph.D., M.S.W., M.P.H.
Executive Director, Silver's McSilver Institute for Poverty Policy and Research
New York University

Joseph Simonetti, M.D., M.P.H.
Physician and Suicide Prevention Researcher,
Rocky Mountain Mental Illness Research Education and Clinical Center for VA Suicide Prevention

Ursula Whiteside, Ph.D.
Chief Executive Officer, NowMattersNow.org
Clinical Faculty, University of Washington

Cathleen Willging, Ph.D.
Center Director and Senior Research Scientist
Pacific Institute for Research and Evaluation
Southwest Center

CLOSING REMARKS

3:25 PM   Michael F. Hogan, Ph.D.
Principal
Hogan Health Solutions LLC
Planning Committee Member

3:30 PM   ADJOURN

PART 2
BUILDING 9-8-8: AN OPPORTUNITY TO BUILD INCLUSIVE CARE STRUCTURES
WEDNESDAY, JULY 28, 2021
11:00 AM–1:30 PM ET

WELCOME FROM THE FORUM ON MENTAL HEALTH AND SUBSTANCE USE DISORDERS

11:00 AM   Mary Roary, Ph.D.
Director, Office of Behavioral Health Equity Office of Intergovernmental and External Affairs
Office of the Assistant Secretary for Mental Health and Substance Use
Substance Abuse and Mental Health Services Administration
Planning Committee Co-Chair

WHY CRISIS SERVICES MUST BE IMPROVED

11:05 AM   Mary Ann Nihart, M.A., APRN, PMHCNS-BC, PMHNP-BC
Associate Director for Patient Care Services, Nurse Executive
San Francisco VA Health Care System

APPENDIX B 83

SESSION 3
THE 9-8-8 LIFELINE: POTENTIAL AND IMPLICATIONS FOR CRISIS RESPONSE

11:15 AM *Session 3 Moderator:*
Erin Bagalman, M.S.W.
Director, Division of Behavioral Health Policy
Office of Behavioral Health, Disability, and Aging Policy
Office of the Assistant Secretary for Planning and Evaluation
U.S. Department of Health and Human Services
Planning Committee Member

Speakers:
Anita Everett, M.D., DFAPA
Director
Center for Mental Health Services
Substance Abuse and Mental Health Services Administration

Richard McKeon, Ph.D.
Chief, Suicide Prevention Branch
Division of Prevention, Traumatic Stress, and Special Programs
Center for Mental Health Services
Substance Abuse and Mental Health Services Administration

Madelyn S. Gould, Ph.D., M.P.H.
Irving Philips Professor of Epidemiology in Psychiatry, Vagelos College of Physicians and Surgeons
Columbia University
Research Scientist
New York State Psychiatric Institute

Lisa Kearney, Ph.D., ABPP
Director, Veterans Crisis Line
Office of Mental Health and Suicide Prevention
U.S. Department of Veterans Affairs

SESSION 4
9-8-8 ROLLOUT: PRIVACY, CONFIDENTIALITY, AND EQUITY CONSIDERATIONS

11:35 AM *Session 4 Moderator:*
Matt Tierney, M.S., APRN
President, American Psychiatric Nurses Association
Clinical Professor, University of California, San Francisco, School of Nursing
Clinical Director of Substance Use Treatment and Education
University of California, San Francisco, Office of Population Health
Planning Committee Co-Chair

Speakers:
Sue Ann O'Brien, LPC, M.B.A.
Chief Executive Officer
Behavioral Health Link

Pamela End of Horn, M.S.W., LICSW
National Suicide Prevention Consultant, Division of Behavioral Health
Office of Clinical and Preventive Services
Indian Health Service

Victor Armstrong, M.S.W.
Director
Division of Mental Health, Developmental Disabilities and Substance Abuse Services
North Carolina Department of Health and Human Services

SESSION 5
BUILDING CULTURAL COMPETENCE WITHIN CRISIS SERVICES

11:50 AM *Session 5 Moderator:*
Jane Pearson, Ph.D.
Special Advisor to the Director on Suicide Research
National Institute of Mental Health
Planning Committee Member

Speakers:
May Yeh, Ph.D.
Associate Professor, Department of Psychology College of Sciences
San Diego State University

Pamela End of Horn, M.S.W., LICSW
National Suicide Prevention Consultant, Division of Behavioral Health
Office of Clinical and Preventive Services
Indian Health Service

Jennifer Battle, M.S.W.
Director of Access
The Harris Center for Mental Health and Intellectual/Developmental Disabilities

Thomas Chávez, Ph.D.
Associate Professor, Counseling Psychology College of Education
Transdisciplinary Research, Equity, Engagement Center
University of New Mexico

Xinzhi Zhang
Chief, Health Inequities and Global Health Branch
Center for Translation Research & Implementation Science
National Heart, Lung, and Blood Institute
National Institutes of Health

Brandon Johnson, M.H.S., MCHES
Public Health Advisor
Center for Mental Health Services
Division of Prevention, Traumatic Stress, and Special Programs Suicide Prevention Branch
Substance Abuse and Mental Health Services Administration

12:20 PM   **BREAK (5 mins)**

12:25 PM   **Brandon Johnson, M.H.S., MCHES**
Public Health Advisor
Center for Mental Health Services
Division of Prevention, Traumatic Stress, and Special Programs
  Suicide Prevention Branch
Substance Abuse and Mental Health Services Administration

Sam Brinton
Vice President of Advocacy and Government Affairs
The Trevor Project

Tracie Schneider, Ed.D., CRC
Division of Aging, Adult, and Behavioral Health Services Deaf
  Services Coordinator
Arkansas Department of Health and Human Services

Sharon Hoover, Ph.D.
Professor, Division of Child and Adolescent Psychiatry
Co-Director, National Center for School Mental Health
Director, National Center for Safe Supportive Schools
University of Maryland School of Medicine

AUDIENCE Q&A

12:50 PM   *Moderator:*
Jane Pearson, Ph.D.
Special Advisor to the Director on Suicide Research
National Institute of Mental Health
Planning Committee Member

ALL SPEAKERS
REFLECTIONS AND OPPORTUNITIES IN BUILDING INCLUSIVE CARE STRUCTURES

1:20 PM   **Barbara Limandri, Ph.D., PMHCNS-BS**
Psychiatric Nurse
American Psychiatric Nurses Association

David Covington, LPC, M.B.A.
Chief Executive Officer and President
RI International Partner
Behavioral Health Link

1:30 PM   **ADJOURN**

Appendix C

Speaker and Moderator Biographies

Victor Armstrong, M.S.W., joined the North Carolina Department of Health and Human Services as the director of the North Carolina Division of Mental Health, Developmental Disabilities, Substance Abuse Services in March 2020, with responsibility and oversight of the public community-based mental health, intellectual and other developmental disabilities, substance use, and traumatic brain injury system in North Carolina. Prior to accepting this role, Armstrong spent 6 years as the vice president of behavioral health with Atrium Health. Based in Charlotte, North Carolina, Armstrong had responsibility for operations of Atrium's largest behavioral health hospital, Behavioral Health Charlotte (BHC). The BHC campus contains the Southeast's only psychiatric emergency department, staffed 24/7 with board-certified psychiatrists, as well as 66 inpatient beds, and 10 outpatient programs. Armstrong has more than 30 years of experience in human services, primarily dedicated to building and strengthening community resources to serve individuals living with mental illness. He currently serves on the board of directors for the American Association of Suicidology, the American Foundation for Suicide Prevention of North Carolina, and United Suicide Survivors International. He is also former the board chair of the National Alliance on Mental Illness (NAMI) North Carolina and a member of the National Association of Social Workers. Armstrong is a former member of the board of directors of the National Council for Behavioral Health, i2i Center for Integrative Health, and RI International. His awards and recognitions include Mental Health America's 2021 H. Keith Brunnemer, Jr., Award for "Outstanding Mental Health Leadership," 2019 Black Mental Health Symposium—Mental Health Advocate of the Year, 2019 Atrium Health

Excellence in Diversity & Inclusion Award, 2018 Distinguished Alumni Award from the East Carolina University School of Social Work, *Pride Magazine* 2018 "Best of the Best," i2i Center for Integrative Health 2018 Innovation Award for "Whole Person Care," and 2012 NAMI North Carolina Mental Health Professional of the Year. Armstrong graduated magna cum laude from North Carolina Central University with a bachelor's degree in business management and received an M.S.W. from East Carolina University.

Erin Bagalman, M.S.W., joined the U.S. Department of Health and Human Services' Office of the Assistant Secretary for Planning and Evaluation (ASPE) in 2018. She serves as the director of the Division of Behavioral Health Policy in ASPE's Office of Behavioral Health, Disability, and Aging Policy. In that role, she manages an interdisciplinary team focused on policies addressing mental health, substance use, and related topics such as suicide. Previously, Bagalman served as the lead analyst for behavioral health policy at the Congressional Research Service, providing non-partisan analysis of behavioral health services, financing, and research. Before that, she worked in the private sector conducting health outcomes research. Bagalman began her career as a psychiatric social worker. She holds a B.A. in political science from the University of Massachusetts Amherst and an M.S.W. from Tulane University.

Jennifer Battle, M.S.W., is the director of access at The Harris Center for Mental Health and Intellectual/Developmental Disabilities (IDD) in Houston, Texas. Battle oversees the Harris Center Access Hub, which includes the Access Line and the Crisis Line that serves as the crisis line for 39 Texas counties as well as a regional provider of the National Suicide Prevention Lifeline, soon to be 9-8-8. She also oversees the Southeast Texas Regional Suicide Care Support Center and the Harris Center Community Outreach Department. In collaboration with the Houston Police Department, Houston Fire Department, and Houston Emergency Communications Center, she leads the 9-1-1 Crisis Call Diversion Program, the first program of its kind in the United States. Battle also leads the implementation team for the agency's Zero Suicide initiative and serves as an advisory council member on the Mayor's Challenge to Prevent Veteran Suicide. In addition to her work at the Harris Center, Battle serves on the board of the National Association of Crisis Organization Directors. She is the co-chair of the National Suicide Prevention Lifeline Steering Committee, serves on the Clinical Advisory Council for Crisis Text Line and as a Crisis Text Line volunteer, and is a Crisis Center site examiner for the American Association of Suicidology.

Crystal Barksdale, Ph.D., M.P.H., is the acting deputy director and the chief of the Minority Mental Health Research Program at the National Institute of Mental Health's (NIMH's) Office for Disparities Research and Workforce Diversity. She provides guidance and expertise related to research on minority mental health and mental health disparities. Prior to joining NIMH, Barksdale worked at the Substance Abuse and Mental Health Services Administration, where she provided program evaluation leadership and subject-matter expertise on children's mental health projects. Barksdale has also worked on projects focused on disparities in child-serving systems and culturally and linguistically appropriate interventions for at-risk youth and their families. She is a licensed clinical psychologist who maintains a client caseload in private practice.

Jeffrey A. Bridge, Ph.D., is an epidemiologist and the director of the Center for Suicide Prevention and Research in the Abigail Wexner Research Institute at Nationwide Children's Hospital; the Nationwide Foundation Endowed Chair of Innovation in Behavioral Health Research; and a professor of pediatrics, psychiatry, and behavioral health at The Ohio State University College of Medicine. His research focuses on the epidemiology of suicide and suicidal behavior in young people, neurocognitive vulnerability to suicidal behavior, screening for suicide risk in medical and school settings, and improving the quality of care and outcomes for suicidal youth.

Lisa A. Brenner, Ph.D., is a board-certified rehabilitation psychologist, a professor of physical medicine and rehabilitation (PM&R), psychiatry, and neurology at the University of Colorado Anschutz Medical Campus, and the director of the U.S. Department of Veterans Affairs Rocky Mountain Mental Illness Research, Education, and Clinical Center (MIRECC). She is also the vice chair of research for the Department of PM&R. Brenner is the past president of Division 22 (Rehabilitation Psychology) of the American Psychological Association (APA) and an APA Fellow. She serves as an associate editor of the *Journal of Head Trauma Rehabilitation*. Her primary area of research interest is traumatic brain injury, comorbid psychiatric disorders, and negative psychiatric outcomes including suicide. Brenner has numerous peer-reviewed publications, participates on national advisory boards, and recently co-authored the book *Suicide Prevention After Neurodisability: An Evidence-Informed Approach*.

Sam Brinton is the vice president of advocacy and government affairs for The Trevor Project, the world's largest suicide prevention and crisis intervention organization for LGBTQ youth. They are the founder of Trevor's 50 Bill 50 States campaign to end the dangerous and discredited practice of conversion therapy, first in the United States and then around the globe. As a survivor of conversion therapy, Brinton has spoken before the United Nations and Congress and testified on legislation from coast to coast to protect LGBTQ youth mental health. Brinton also led the federal legislative campaign leading to the passage of the National Suicide Hotline Designation Act, the nation's first unanimously supported LGBTQ-inclusive legislation. They have been featured in numerous media including multiple *The New York Times* op-eds and *The Washington Post*, *Playboy* Magazine, and *TIME* Magazine. Sam uses they, them, or their pronouns as a gender-fluid person.

Thomas Anthony Chávez is an assistant professor and research faculty at the University of New Mexico (UNM). Upon graduating from the University of Wisconsin–Madison in counseling psychology, he provided clinical service and taught counselor education to diverse communities. His scholarly work explores social determinants of Latinx health, healing, and wellness through community-engaged approaches. He has received National Institutes of Health grant funding through the UNM Transdisciplinary Research on Equity and Engagement Center to explore the experiences of undocumented Latinx individuals and families.

David W. Covington, LPC, M.B.A., is the chief executive officer and president of Recovery Innovations, Inc. (RI International). He is a behavioral health innovator, entrepreneur and storyteller. He is also a partner in Behavioral Health Link and the founder of the international innovations "Moving America's Soul on Suicide," "Zero Suicide," "Crisis Now," "Crisis Talk" and "Hope Inc. Stories." A licensed professional counselor, Covington received an M.B.A. from Kennesaw State and an M.S. from the University of Memphis. He previously served as the vice president at Magellan Health, where he was responsible for the executive and clinical operations of the $750 million Arizona contract. He is a member of the U.S. Department of Health and Human Services' Interdepartmental Serious Mental Illness Coordinating Committee, which was established in 2017 in accordance with the 21st Century Cures Act to report to Congress on advances in behavioral health. Covington is a two-time national winner of the Council of State Governments Innovations Award (2008 and 2012). He also competed as a finalist in Harvard's Innovations in American Government in 2009 for the Georgia Crisis and Access Line, and the program was featured in *BusinessWeek* magazine. Covington has served on the National Action Alliance for Suicide Prevention Executive Committee since 2010. He was also the vice chair of the National Suicide Prevention Lifeline Substance Abuse and Mental Health Services Administration Steering Committee from 2005 until 2020 and served as a former president of the American Association of Suicidology. He has served on numerous committees and task forces on clinical care and crisis services, including the National Council for Behavioral Health Board of Directors.

Pamela End of Horn, M.S.W., LICSW, is responsible for the development and oversight of the Suicide Prevention and Care Program at the Indian

Health Service. Her work focuses on program policy development, program implementation, and evaluation. End of Horn has an M.S.W. and currently holds advanced practice licenses in North Dakota and Minnesota. End of Horn is an enrolled member of the Oglala Lakota Sioux of the Pine Ridge Indian Reservation, Pine Ridge, South Dakota. She is currently completing a doctorate in social work at the University of Pennsylvania.

Anita Smith Everett, M.D., DFAPA, currently serves as the director of the Center for Mental Health Services in the Substance Abuse and Mental Health Services Administration (SAMHSA). There she oversees the administration of grants that aim to increase mental health literacy and build responsive mental health services for crises management, ongoing treatment, and recovery support for children and adults. Everett comes to SAMHSA with extensive experience in the delivery and leadership of psychiatric services for persons with schizophrenia and other psychiatric conditions in health underserved areas. Previously she was faculty in the Department of Psychiatry at Johns Hopkins University School of Medicine and Bloomberg School of Public Health. She is a past president of the American Psychiatric Association, the American Association of Community Psychiatrists, and has received commendation for her work in national health care reform and advocacy.

Madelyn Gould, Ph.D., M.P.H., is the Irving Philips Professor of Epidemiology in Psychiatry at the Columbia University Medical Center in the United States and a research scientist at the New York State Psychiatric Institute, where she directs the Community Suicide Prevention Research Group. For nearly four decades, she has attained international recognition as an expert in the area of suicide prevention, conducting numerous federally funded grants from the National Institute of Health, the Centers for Disease Control and Prevention, and the Substance Abuse and Mental Health Services Administration (SAMHSA), as well as collaborating on research studies with international investigators, and publishing several seminal articles on youth suicide risk and preventive interventions. Gould has a strong commitment to applying her research to program and policy development. Her current projects focus on the evaluation of suicide crisis interventions via telephone, chat, and text. This research has been used by SAMHSA and the National Suicide Prevention Lifeline to support the passage of the National Suicide Hotline Designation Act of 2020. Her research—most notably in the areas of suicide contagion/clusters; screening and assessment of suicide risk; and crisis interventions—has laid the groundwork for state, national, and international suicide prevention programs. Her research contributions have been recognized by numerous awards, including the Shneidman Award for Research from the American Association of Suicidology (AAS), the New York State (NYS) Office of Mental Health Research

Award, the American Foundation for Suicide Prevention Research Award, the NYS Suicide Prevention Center's Excellence in Suicide Prevention Award, and the Dublin Award from AAS, which is a lifetime achievement award for outstanding contributions to the field of suicide prevention.

Michael Hogan, Ph.D., served as the New York State (NYS) commissioner of mental health from 2007 to 2012, and now operates a consulting practice in health and behavioral health care. The NYS Office of Mental Health operated 23 accredited psychiatric hospitals and oversaw New York's $5 billion public mental health system serving 650,000 individuals annually. Previously Hogan served as the director of the Ohio Department of Mental Health (1991–2007) and as the commissioner of the Connecticut State Department of Mental Health and Addiction Services from 1987 to 1991. He chaired the president's New Freedom Commission on Mental Health in 2002–2003. He served as the first behavioral health representative on the board of The Joint Commission (2007–2015) and chaired its Standards and Survey Procedures Committee. He has served as a member of the National Action Alliance for Suicide Prevention since it was created in 2010, co-chairing task forces on clinical care, interventions, and crisis care. Previously, he served on the National Institute of Mental Health Council (1994–1998 and 2014–2018), as the president of the National Association of State Mental Health Program Directors (2003–2005) and as the board president of the National Association of State Mental Health Program Director's Research Institute (1989–2000). His awards for national leadership include recognition by the National Governors Association, the National Alliance on Mental Illness, and the Campaign for Mental Health Reform, the American College of Mental Health Administration, and the American Psychiatric Association. He is a graduate of Cornell University (B.S., 1960), and earned an M.S. from the State University College in Brockport, New York (1972), and a Ph.D. from Syracuse University (1977).

Sharon A. Hoover, Ph.D., is a licensed clinical psychologist and a professor in the Division of Child and Adolescent Psychiatry,at the University of Maryland School of Medicine and the co-director of the National Center for School Mental Health (www.schoolmentalhealth.org). She currently leads national efforts to support states, districts, and schools in the adoption of national performance standards of comprehensive school mental health systems (www.theSHAPEsystem.com). Hoover has led and collaborated on multiple federal and state grants, with a commitment to the study and implementation of quality children's mental health services. Creating safe, supportive, and resilient schools has been a major emphasis of Hoover's research, education, and clinical work. She has worked with the National Child Traumatic Stress Network (NCTSN) to train school district and school leaders, educators, and support staff in multi-tiered systems of support for psychological trauma. She has trained school and community behavioral health staff and educators in districts across the United States and internationally. In 2020, Hoover was awarded a Substance Abuse and Mental Health Services Administration grant to develop the NCTSN Center for Safe Supportive Schools (www.ncs3.org), aimed at integrating trauma-informed policies and practices in school mental health systems, with a specific focus on social justice and supporting youth of color, newcomer youth, and other marginalized students and families. Since the onset of COVID-19, Hoover has worked with education and mental health leaders across the United States as they support educators, students, and their families with social, emotional, and academic needs amid the global pandemic.

Brandon J. Johnson, M.H.S., MCHES, is a tireless advocate for positive mental health and suicide prevention services for youth and adults across the country. Johnson earned a B.S. from Morgan State University in 2008 and an M.H.S. from Johns Hopkins University in 2012. Currently, he serves as a public health advisor at the Substance Abuse Mental Health Services Administration in the Suicide Prevention Branch at the U.S. Department of Health and Human Services. In this role, Johnson serves as a government project officer (GPO) for various suicide prevention grant programs that respectively target youth, adults, and health care systems. Johnson is the program lead of the Garrett Lee Smith State/Tribal Suicide Prevention Program, which provides grants for states, tribes, and territories to reduce suicides among 10- to 24-year-olds. He is also the GPO for the Suicide Prevention Resource Center, which provides suicide-specific materials, webinars, and training to organizations and communities all over the country working to prevent suicides. Another highlight of Johnson's career is his current role as the co-lead of the National Action Alliance for Suicide Prevention's Faith Communities Task Force. The group works with faith communities all over the nation to equip them with tools and resources to combat the often stigmatized issue of suicide. He serves as the subject-matter expert in suicide among Black people and has lead numerous projects to develop resources and materials to specifically prevent suicide among African American youth. Previously, Johnson served as the director of suicide and violence prevention for the State of Maryland, where he worked in communities throughout the state to help develop strategies to end violence in various forms, such as community violence and human trafficking.

Lisa K. Kearney, Ph.D., ABPP, provides oversight to the development and implementation of the U.S. Department of Veterans Affairs' (VA's) comprehensive public health approach to suicide prevention, combining both community-based prevention and clinically based intervention strategies. She is responsible for overseeing the day-to-day operations of the Suicide Prevention Program and the Veterans Crisis Line, which provides 24/7 crisis line support to veterans and service members through calls, chat, and text services. Kearney recently served as the deputy director of suicide prevention and the associate director of education at the VA Center for Integrated Healthcare. Previously, she worked nationally as part of the executive team in the VA Office of Mental Health Operations as the senior consultant for technical assistance, overseeing mental health policy implementation through quality improvement site visits across the VA system. At the local level, Kearney served as the chief of psychology, assistant chief, director of training, and director of primary care mental health integration at the South Texas Veterans Health Care System. Kearney is also a clinical associate professor of psychiatry at the University of Texas Health Science Center in San Antonio. She is the associate editor for *Psychological Services* and an editor for *Psychology of Men and Masculinity*. She currently serves as the past president of the American Academy of Clinical Health Psychology. She has received the following national awards: American Psychological Association (APA) Excellence in Clinical Health Psychology Award (2020), Association of Psychologists in Academic Health Centers Outstanding Mid-Career Professional Contributions Award (2019), Russell B. Lemle Leadership Award (2018), APA Presidential Citation (2016), APA Peter J. N. Linnerooth National Service Award (2015), and Association of VA Psychologist Leaders Special Contribution Award (2010). She is a fellow in APA Division 18, APA Division 38, the American Academy of Clinical Health Psychology, and the Bexar County Psychological Association. She is an active member of the American Psychological Association, the American Academy of Clinical Health Psychology, and the Association of VA Psychologist Leaders, and has more than 40 publications in the areas of integrated primary care, suicide prevention, mental health business operations, and training of mental health providers.

Barbara Limandri, Ph.D., PMHNP, BC, is a retired psychiatric mental health nurse practitioner and a professor emerita at Linfield University in Portland, Oregon. She earned her baccalaureate degree in nursing at Virginia Commonwealth University, her master's degree in psychiatric-mental health nursing at The Catholic University of America, and her doctorate in psychiatric nursing at the University of California, San Francisco. She is a member of the American Psychiatric Nurses Association (APNA) where she co-chaired the task force to develop clinical competencies for psychiatric nurses for suicide prevention and management. As a follow-up on those competencies, Limandri co-chaired the committee to develop a curriculum to prepare nurses to meet those competences and has taught more than 20 workshops throughout the United States in suicide prevention and management. Additionally, Limandri helped develop the training course for facilitators of the Suicide Prevention

Training workshop and has taught the course for 5 years for APNA. Limandri has authored several articles related to suicide prevention and two textbook chapters. In addition, Limandri has expertise in Dialectical Behavior Therapy (DBT) that was originally developed to assist those struggling with chronic suicidal thinking and behavior associated with borderline personality disorder. Treatment strategies used in DBT includes individual psychotherapy, skill development in groups, and pharmacotherapy.

Michael A. Lindsey, Ph.D., M.S.W., M.P.H., is a noted scholar in the fields of child and adolescent mental health and a leader in the search for knowledge and solutions to generational poverty and inequality. He is the executive director of the McSilver Institute for Poverty Policy and Research at New York University (NYU), the Constance and Martin Silver Professor of Poverty Studies at the NYU Silver School of Social Work, and an Aspen Health Innovators Fellow. He also leads a university-wide Strategies to Reduce Inequality initiative from the NYU McSilver Institute. At the McSilver Institute, Lindsey leads a team of researchers, clinicians, social workers, and other professionals who are committed to creating new knowledge about the root causes of poverty, developing evidence-based interventions to address its consequences, and rapidly translating their findings into action through policy and best practices. Additionally, he leads the working group of experts supporting the Congressional Black Caucus Emergency Taskforce on Black Youth Suicide and Mental Health, which created the report *Ring the Alarm: The Crisis of Black Youth Suicide in America*. Lindsey is a Distinguished Fellow of the National Academies of Practice in Social Work, and serves on the editorial boards of *Administration and Policy in Mental Health and Mental Health Services Research*, the *Journal of Clinical Child and Adolescent Psychology*, *Psychiatric Services*, *School Mental Health*, and *Prevention Science*. He holds a Ph.D. in social work, an M.P.H. from the University of Pittsburgh, an M.S.W. from Howard University, and a B.A. in sociology from Morehouse College.

Richard McKeon, Ph.D., M.P.H., received his Ph.D. in clinical psychology from the University of Arizona, and an M.P.H. in health administration from Columbia University. He has spent most of his career working in community mental health, including 11 years as the director of a psychiatric emergency service and 4 years as the associate administrator/clinical director of a hospital-based community mental health center in Newton, New Jersey. In 2001, he was awarded an American Psychological Association Congressional Fellowship and worked in the U.S. Senate, covering health and mental health policy issues. He spent 5 years on the Board of the American Association of Suicidology as the clinical division director and has also served on the Board of the Division of Clinical Psychology of the American Psychological Association.

He is currently the chief for the Suicide Prevention Branch in the Center for Mental Health Services of the Substance Abuse and Mental Health Services Administration, where he oversees all branch suicide prevention activities, including the Garrett Lee Smith State/Tribal Youth Suicide Prevention, and Campus Suicide Prevention grant programs, the National Suicide Prevention Lifeline, the Suicide Prevention Resource Center, and the Native Connections program. In 2008, he was appointed by the Secretary of the U.S. Department of Veterans Affairs to the Secretary's Blue Ribbon Work Group on Suicide Prevention. In 2009, he was appointed by the Secretary of the U.S. Department of Defense to its Task Force on Suicide Prevention in the Military. He served on the National Action Alliance for Suicide Prevention Task Force that revised the National Strategy for Suicide Prevention and participated in the development of the World Health Organization's World Suicide Prevention Report. He is also the co-chair of the Federal Working Group on Suicide Prevention.

Mary Ann Nihart, M.A., APRN, PMHCNS-BC, PMHNP-BC, currently serves as the associate director for patient care services and the nurse executive at the San Francisco Veterans Affairs (VA) Healthcare System. Despite her primarily administrative role, Nihart continues to practice as a psychiatric mental health nurse practitioner. She established the first PMHNP residency program at the San Francisco VA in conjunction with the University of California, San Francisco, where she is an associate clinical professor in the School of Nursing. She is a nationally and internationally known speaker as an early integrator of biology in psychiatric mental health nursing and has spent much of her career developing and working with community agencies on crisis management. Nihart also served as the mayor of the City of Pacifica. She was also the president-elect of the American Psychiatric Nurses Association (APNA) and one of the most recent award winners of the APNA Psychiatric Nurse of the Year.

Sue Ann O'Brien, LPC, M.B.A., is the president and the chief executive officer (CEO) at Behavioral Health Link (BHL) and the executive vice president at RI International. Together, these two teams deliver a full continuum of best practice crisis services, powered by customized software and technology solutions and real-time access to mental health and substance use services, diverting thousands from hospital emergency departments and justice systems to care in communities throughout the United States. They were both leading contributors to the development of the National Action Alliance for Suicide Prevention's Crisis Now exceptional practice standards in crisis care. As the CEO of BHL, O'Brien leads a team of visionary crisis innovators whose breakthrough technology and crisis services have been featured worldwide. Recognized for innovation by the National Council for Behavioral Health, the Council of State Governments, Harvard University, and others, BHL operates Georgia's statewide Crisis and Access Line, offering the nation's broadest application of advanced crisis call center technology through its Care Traffic Control system. BHL also delivers and/or deploys 24/7 community-based mobile crisis in all 159 Georgia counties. O'Brien was formerly the chief operating officer at RI International and was previously responsible for Crisis Facility services spanning five states. RI, which founded the "living room" model in 2002, deliver no-wrong-door, facility-based crisis services in seven states with rapid growth targeted. RI's Campus of Connection model includes a strong peer workforce and surrounds the individual with support on their journey toward recovery. With 25 years of senior leadership experience in behavioral health, O'Brien aims to foster and create crisis care equivalents to the nation's rapid response system for individuals with medical emergencies by making care available to anyone, anywhere, and anytime. Together, these two strategic partners employ nearly 1,800 staff and have offices in Arizona, California, Delaware, Georgia, Louisiana (2020), New Zealand, North Carolina, Virginia (2020), and Washington State, and their impact is growing through consulting, training, and crisis immersion experiences.

Jane Pearson, Ph.D., is a widely recognized authority on suicide and suicide prevention with expertise in clinical psychology and public health strategies. She serves as the special advisor to the director of the National Institute of Mental Health (NIMH) on suicide research. She leads the NIMH Suicide Research Team and serves on the National Action Alliance for Suicide Prevention Research Task Force. She assisted in the development of the first Surgeon General's Call to Action to Prevent Suicide and the first U.S. National Strategy for Suicide Prevention. Pearson is also an adjunct associate professor at Johns Hopkins University and a fellow of the American Psychological Association. She has practiced as a licensed clinical psychologist and has authored papers on the ethical and methodological challenges of suicide research.

Mary Roary, Ph.D., is a public health epidemiologist who focuses on infectious and chronic diseases. Roary is currently the director of the Office of Behavioral Health Equity at the Substance Abuse and Mental Health Services Administration. She is also an adjunct professor at The Catholic University of America. She has worked across government, academia, and the private industry. Roary has worked in two components of the National Institutes of Health (NIH) since 2013 as a program director and an officer. At NIH, Roary was responsible for health promotion, disease prevention, environmental influences, health disparities, low resources in the "IDeA States," and child health portfolio. Roary has developed national funding opportunities, overseen complex budgets, mentored investigators in developing project grants, and disseminated research findings to stakeholders. Roary previously served as the data lead for the U.S. Department of Health and Human Services' Office of Minority Health Committees on the Patient Protection and Affordable Care Act, Healthy People 2020, and environmental justice. She was the principal investigator and co-principal investigator for multiple community-based participatory research grants at Johns Hopkins University and the University of Arizona. Roary earned her Ph.D. in epidemiology and was an epidemiology and biostatistician Centers for Disease Control and Prevention fellow at the University of Arizona. She holds several master's degrees from Johns Hopkins University. Her ultimate goal is to become an influential champion of eliminating health disparities by identifying and implementing data-driven best practices that promote health equity and wellness.

Tracie Schneider, Ed.D., CRC, has worked in the intersection of disability, employment, and education for more than 10 years. She currently serves as Arkansas' Department of Human Services deaf mental health coordinator. Her background is in accessibility, policy development, service coordination, and vocational rehabilitation counseling. She earned her bachelor's degree from Texas A&M University in Texarkana, Texas; her master's degree from Southern University and A&M College in Baton Rouge, Louisiana; and her doctorate from Lamar University in Beaumont, Texas. Her primary areas of interest are deaf mental health, communication equity, and transition services for youth with disabilities.

Joseph Simonetti, M.D., M.P.H., earned his M.D. from The Ohio State University and completed his training in internal medicine at the University of Pittsburgh. He then completed an National Research Service Award health services research fellowship, worked as a senior research fellow at the Harborview Injury Prevention & Research Center at the University of Washington and the U.S. Department of Veterans Affairs' (VA's) Patient-Aligned Care Team National Demonstration Lab, and he earned and M.P.H. from the University of Washington School of Public Health. Currently, he is an internal medicine physician practicing within the VA Eastern Colorado Healthcare System. He has research appointments within the VA Rocky Mountain Mental Illness Research, Education and Clinical Center for Suicide Prevention and the Denver-Seattle Center of Innovation for Veteran-Centered and Value-Driven Care. Simonetti's research focuses on reducing the burden of intentional and unintentional firearm injuries nationally. His current focus is on creating infrastructure for stakeholder engagement in firearm-related research, and developing veteran-centered approaches to facilitating lethal means safety as a suicide prevention strategy.

Matthew Tierney, M.S., APRN, is a clinical professor at the UCSF School of Nursing and is clinical director of substance use treatment and education for the Office of Population Health at UCSF Health. He is currently the president of the American Psychiatric Nurses Association (APNA) and represents APNA on the National Academies' Forum on Mental Health and Substance Use Disorders. An educator and a clinician for more than two decades, his work focuses on increasing access to essential mental health and substance use treatment by developing and implementing innovative clinical treatment programs and by educating the existing and rising health care workforce. As an active nurse practitioner certified in adult primary care, addictions nursing, and psychiatric-mental health care, his clinical work focuses on providing evidence-based care to vulnerable and highly stigmatized populations. He is an active participant in numerous professional organizations including the Association for Multidisciplinary Education and Research in Substance use and Addiction; the American Society of Addiction Medicine (ASAM), where he serves on the national Planning Committee for the Treatment of Opioid Use Disorder Course Program; and ASAM's California Chapter (CSAM) where he serves as the only nurse on the Committee on Opioids and as an educator and a mentor in CSAM's Medical Education and Research Foundation. He is also a fellow of the American Academy of Nursing where he actively serves on the Expert Panel on Psychiatric-Mental Health and Substance Use.

Ursula Whiteside, Ph.D., is a licensed clinical psychologist, the chief executive officer of NowMattersNow.org, and clinical faculty at the University of Washington. As a researcher, she has been awarded grants from the National Institute of Mental Health (NIMH) and the American Foundation for Suicide Prevention. Clinically, she began her training with Dr. Marsha Linehan in 1999 and later served as a Dialectical Behavior Therapy (DBT)-adherent research therapist on an NIMH-funded clinical trial led by Dr. Linehan. Whiteside is a group- and individual-certified DBT clinician. Now, she treats high-risk suicidal clients in her small private practice in Seattle using DBT and caring contacts. Whiteside is national faculty for the Zero Suicide initiative, a practical approach to suicide prevention in health care and behavioral health care systems. This program was described by NPR on a segment titled "What Happens If You Try to Prevent Every Single Suicide?" She is also the vice president of United Suicide Survivors International. As a person with lived experience, she strives to decrease the gap between "us and them" and to ensure that the voices of those who have been there are included in all relevant conversations: nothing about us without us.

Holly Wilcox, Ph.D., is a professor in the Department of Mental Health at the Johns Hopkins Bloomberg School of Public Health with joint appointments in the Department of Health Policy and Management and the Johns

Hopkins University Schools of Medicine and Education. Much of her work involves population-based research on suicide, intergenerational studies of suicide, the evaluation of the impact of community-based universal prevention programs, and data linkage strategies to inform suicide prevention. Wilcox leads a multidisciplinary, interdepartmental suicide prevention work group at Johns Hopkins University. She has a diverse publication history that demonstrates her experience in biological, psychological, and social factors in suicide. Wilcox was appointed by Governor Larry Hogan to the Maryland School Board. She also co-chairs the Maryland Commission on Suicide Prevention. She has twice received the Johns Hopkins Bloomberg School of Public Health's Excellence in Advising, Mentoring, Teaching and Research Advising award.

Cathleen Willging, Ph.D., is a medical anthropologist and a senior research scientist at the Pacific Institute for Research and Evaluation with experience in mixed-method research, intervention development and evaluation, and implementation science. Her research focuses on public mental health and substance use treatment in the United States, health care reform, evidence-based practice implementation and sustainment in complex systems, and the advancement of culturally and contextually relevant programs to support marginalized groups affected by inequities. Her current work entails the application of implementation science theory and methods to support innovative programming to reduce health and health care disparities for minoritized populations in diverse service delivery settings, such as primary care practices, hospital emergency departments, and educational institutions. She is especially interested in using participatory methods to promote community engagement in the dissemination, uptake, and sustainment of effective interventions at the individual, organization, and systems levels.

May Yeh, Ph.D., is an associate professor of psychology at San Diego State University (SDSU), a research scientist at the Child and Adolescent Services Research Center; an associate adjunct professor of psychiatry at the University of California, San Diego; and a member of the faculty in the SDSU/University of California, San Diego, joint doctoral program in clinical psychology. Her work focuses on cultural issues, cultural competence, and personalization of evidence-based treatment in mental health services for children.

Xinzhi Zhang, M.D., Ph.D., FACE, is the chief of health inequities and the Global Health Branch at the Center for Translation Research and Implementation Science at the National Heart, Lung, and Blood Institute (NHLBI), part of the National Institutes of Health (NIH). Zhang has broad research interests that include clinical epidemiology, health services research, data science,